cycle savvy

D0404767

ALSO BY TONI WESCHLER

Taking Charge of Your Fertility:
The Definitive Guide to Natural Birth Control,
Pregnancy Achievement, and Reproductive Health

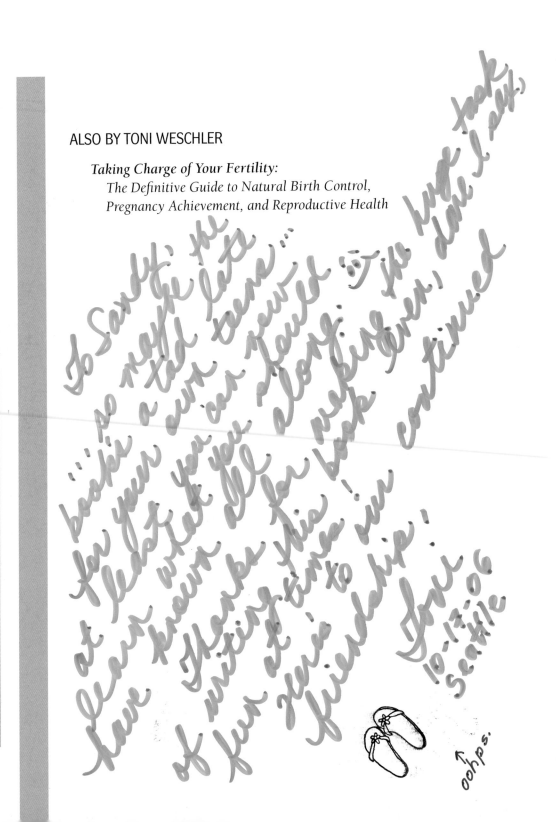

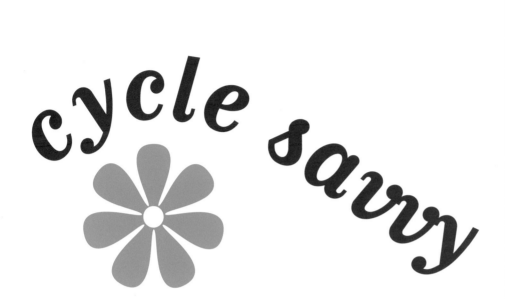

cycle savvy

The Smart Teen's Guide
to the Mysteries of Her Body

Toni Weschler, MPH

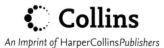

Collins

An Imprint of HarperCollinsPublishers

Disclaimer

This book contains information relating to health care. It is not intended to replace medical advice and should be used to supplement rather than replace regular care by your doctor. It is recommended that you seek your physician's advice before embarking on any medical program or treatment.

All efforts have been made to ensure the accuracy of the information contained in this book as of the date published. The author and the publisher expressly disclaim responsibility for any adverse effect arising from the use or application of the information contained herein.

The names and identifying characteristics of individuals featured throughout this book have been changed to protect their privacy.

CYCLE SAVVY. Copyright © 2006 by Toni Weschler, MPH. All rights reserved. Printed in the United States of America. No part of this book may be used or reproduced in any manner whatsoever without written permission except in the case of the master charts designed for copying at the end of the book, or brief quotations embodied in critical articles and review. For information, address HarperCollins Publishers, 10 East 53rd Street, New York, NY 10022.

Permissions and credits:
Color illustrations by Neil Jeffery
Medical illustrations by Kate Sweeney
Illustration at top of page 4 by Rosy Aronson

HarperCollins books may be purchased for educational, business, or sales promotional use. For information please write: Special Markets Department, HarperCollins Publishers, 10 East 53rd Street, New York, NY 10022.

FIRST EDITION

Designed by Jaime Putorti

Library of Congress Cataloging-in-Publication Data has been applied for.

ISBN-10: 0-06-082964-8
ISBN-13: 978-0-06-082964-3

06 07 08 09 10   WBC/RRD   10 9 8 7 6 5 4 3 2 1

Dedicated with love to my two wonderful nieces,
Sara and Sabrina Weschler,
with hopes that they grow into healthy and confident young women

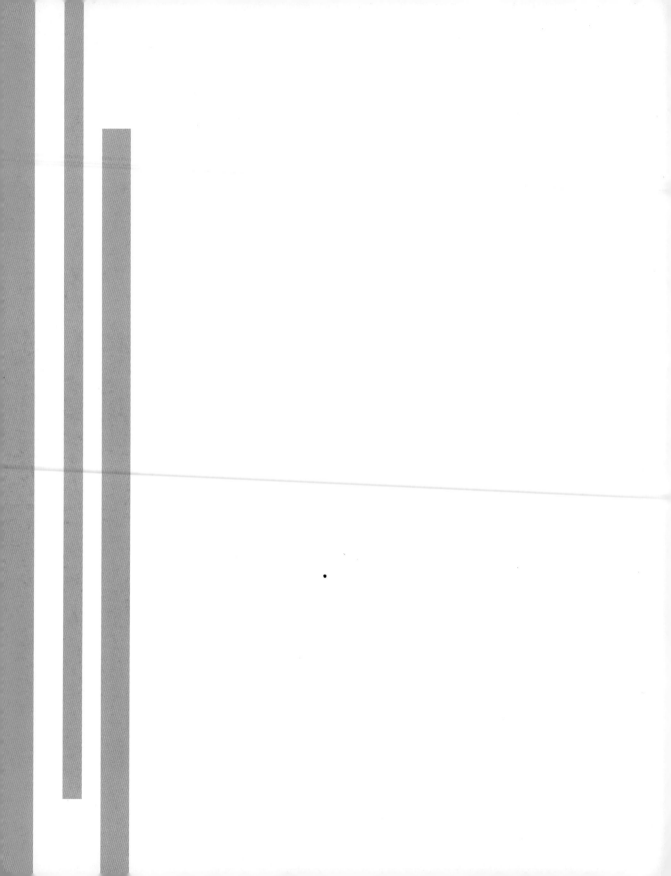

contents

Appendixes

acknowledgments

What was I thinking? After ten years and boxes of letters since the publication of my first book, *Taking Charge of Your Fertility (TCOYF)*, I finally caved in. Me, the wiped-out-from-the-first-book author who claimed she would never take on such an intimidating project again. So what convinced me to write another book, after all? All those women whose correspondence fill those boxes!

The most consistent feedback I've gotten since *TCOYF*'s release continues to reflect a theme along the lines of "Why didn't they teach us this when we were *teenagers*?" or more specifically, "I wish I had known *then* what I know now." After about the zillionth time hearing these comments, I concluded that, you know, maybe my readers were on to something!

It was their letters, so many of which had the same fervent theme running throughout, that ultimately gave me the impetus to tackle such a challenging endeavor. How could I ignore yet one more woman insisting that the next generation of girls have the privilege of growing up with such fundamental and empowering information about their bodies? So to them and all the other wonderful women who so generously contributed stories of their own teenage years in the hopes that it would help girls to make wise and thoughtful decisions that they would never regret, I say thank you.

❋ ❋ ❋

And thanks to my special coterie of six women who had the courage to read my unedited manuscript way before it was ready. Specifically:

To Sandy Sarber, one of the most creative and articulate people I know, for her always-entertaining brainstorming sessions that brought so much levity to an otherwise overwhelming project.

To Cricky Kavanaugh, my incredible assistant on my first book, who continued to bless me with her unwavering support and consistently great ideas.

To Emilie Coulter, one of my very first students in Seattle about 17 years ago, for her sense of humor as she pored over every page (that humor will certainly come in handy now that her newborn daughter, Etta, has arrived on the scene).

To Katja Shaye, my neighbor and friend, for her great ideas and advice.

To Anya Nartker, who had a wonderful knack for balancing sometimes discouraging text with uplifting suggestions.

And to Kimberly Christianson, the midwife of the group, who so often steered me in the right direction with her complete and insightful honesty.

❋ ❋ ❋

To "The Divine Nine," a group of enthusiastic teen girls who all met in Lake Tapps to discuss ways that the book could better help girls learn about their bodies. You all know who you are. You rock!

To Lori Goe, Katrina Harper, and Charlotte Doggett, who all offered me such great suggestions from teenagers' perspectives.

To all the teens who anonymously shared their thoughts and personal stories with me so that others could realize that their own experiences are common to so many girls.

❋ ❋ ❋

To Kate Travers, my former editor at HarperCollins who painstakingly fought for me when *Cycle Savvy* was but a proposal.

To Toni Sciarra, my current editor, and her talented production team of Diane Aronson, Leah Carlson-Stanisic, Susan Kosko, Karen Lumley, Rita Madrigal, Cecilia Molinari, Jaime Putorti, Bill Ruoto, and Donna Ruvituso (phew, it takes a village!), who patiently guided me through the incredible complexities of publishing such a challenging book.

❋ ❋ ❋

To Kyra Butzel, Brangien Davis, Nedra Fekete, and Michal Schonbrun, who helped me untangle some incredibly sticky issues I needed to resolve before even beginning to write.

To Bob Birkby, my fellow author and friend, who saved me from myself when I was going nuts near the end.

To the hundreds of bees who thought it would be kinda funny to build a nest in the wall and invade my office in the midst of my deadlines, for having the courtesy to not sting me as I apprehensively persevered while they buzzed around my head.

❀ ❀ ❀

To Kate Sweeney, my phenomenal medical illustrator, for both this book and my first book, *Taking Charge of Your Fertility*.

To Rosy Aronson, for her gorgeous drawing on page 4, and for always being such a pleasure to work with.

To Neil Jeffery, my incredibly talented and absolutely wonderful illustrator of the charming teen images. I can't thank him enough for his amazing attitude and patience throughout this project. His daughter Jada is very lucky to have him as her daddy.

❀ ❀ ❀

To my dear friend and inspiration, Caroline Dulberg, for her warmth, encouragement, and most of all, incredible sense of humor.

To Roger, who has loyally stood by me with his charming wit while witnessing me have numerous author meltdowns.

To my older brothers Rennie (Lawrence) and Robert and their respective wives Joasia and Jun, for providing me with the inspiration to write this book in the form of two wonderful teenage nieces, Sara and Sabrina (and even a really cool nephew, Sky). And to Wendy, for making my younger brother Raymond so happy and productive.

And finally to Raymond himself who, as with my first book, *Taking Charge*, was absolutely indispensable in writing this one. Again, he was an amazing researcher, editor, organizer, and co-writer. No doubt that such roles were even more of a challenge this time, because he and I had so many, how shall I say, "spirited" debates on how to approach such a tricky subject. Yet, despite all of our differences, it was our incredibly close relationship that ultimately allowed us to produce what we both hope will be a second successful example of genuine sibling teamwork. So to him I offer my greatest appreciation for being such a fantastic brother and one of my best friends.

a note to moms

(AS WELL AS AUNTS, OLDER SISTERS, TEACHERS, AND SCHOOL NURSES)

t en years ago, I wrote the first edition of *Taking Charge of Your Fertility: The Definitive Guide to Natural Birth Control, Pregnancy Achievement and Reproductive Health.* In the years since, I have been thrilled by the growing grassroots movement in Fertility Awareness education that the book has helped to generate across the country.

I've been especially gratified by the hundreds of effusive letters I've received from readers over the years, scores of which questioned why such invaluable and empowering biological information wasn't routinely taught when they were teenagers. For most, this would have been an ideal time to learn about all the gynecological and menstrual enigmas that add so much confusion and insecurity to everyday life, and the knowledge would have prepared them to deal with the inevitable fertility-related issues that they faced later in their adult lives.

Now, lest you start wondering whether this is an appropriate book for your teenage daughter, I should assure you from the start that unlike my first book, which is specifically about the Fertility Awareness *Method*, or FAM, this is *not* a book about how to use effective natural birth control, much less how to get pregnant! However, it is very much a book about the various *fertility signs* that all teen girls have, some of which, like cervical fluid and mid-cycle pain, they are certainly very much aware of, most likely don't understand, and may be too afraid or insecure to ask about.

Of course, there are other signs they may not even realize their bodies produce that most of them would be fascinated to learn about, such as observable patterns in waking temperature and cervical position. Taken as a whole, these various signs serve as an incredibly revealing window into a developing teen's ever-changing body, as well as provide an invaluable sense of bodily confidence, wisdom, and self-esteem that was simply not available to previous generations.

✻ WHAT EVERY TEEN GIRL SHOULD KNOW

This book will not be like the "period pamphlet" that we all received in our junior high school health class. To be sure, perhaps the only menstrual education that most of us ever got in school or even from our own well-intentioned mothers was a solemn accounting of the difference between tampons and sanitary pads, or if they were really trying to enlighten us, some additional wisdom on bras, acne, and feminine hygiene. In fairness, the information we learned was useful for what it was, but ultimately, we were taught virtually nothing practical about the amazing hormonal changes that come with puberty.

Thus, we often had no idea how to react to an endless array of everyday menstrual experiences, from intermittent spotting and sudden sharp abdominal pains to those recurring rounds of vaginal secretions. Adolescence often brought apparently inexplicable mood swings, breast lumps that sometimes caused panic, and for those who were sexually active, constant worry over periods that so often arrived "late."

Well, maybe late, maybe not. Periods are rarely overdue if you know when you actually ovulated, and they, along with most menstrual phenomena, could and should be transformed from being sources of constant anxiety into illuminating and observable signs of a normal cyclical nature. When we were teenagers, these topics were rarely, if ever, taught, much less discussed. But I imagine you would agree that your own teenage daughters deserve much more. I hope that with the help of this book, they will become part of the first generation that's truly "cycle savvy."

❋ THE POWER OF SELF-OBSERVATION

This book is written for girls from about 14 to 18 years old. Since it is generally assumed that a girl this age usually has had her period for a few years, I will skip the basic "what to expect" introduction to early menstrual life and instead will focus on helping a girl to understand the remarkable workings of her continually developing body. She'll master a wealth of self-knowledge by learning to chart her cycles in less than a couple of minutes a day. Through charting, she will soon be able to take control of her own gynecological health, by accurately observing where she is in her cycle, and more specifically, when she has actually ovulated.

As she'll learn, it is *ovulation*, not menstruation, that is the key point of reference in any given cycle, and being able to correctly detect when this occurs each cycle will give her a sense of confidence, feminine self-esteem, and respect for her body that will likely leave you wondering why you couldn't have learned all this yourself, all those years ago. To be sure, knowledge *is* power, and I believe that the information presented in this book is so profoundly practical and empowering that it will one day be seen as a part of every teenage girl's basic health education.

Still, information should always be age appropriate, and thus I want to be very clear again that while this book has everything to do with fertility *awareness*, I have chosen not to present the contraceptive rules of the Fertility Awareness *Method*. Following those rules is, in fact, a highly effective form of natural birth control, based on the scientific principles that your daughter will learn in this book. (Please also note that as such, FAM has nothing to do with the notoriously ineffective rhythm method!)

However, precisely because natural birth control involves no barriers or hormones, *it should only be practiced by very mature and disciplined women who are involved in long-term monogamous relationships.* Yet every teen who masters the material in this book will at least have a major head start in learning the method if she one day so desires, when it would be appropriate to do so. Those contraceptive rules, as well as ways to maximize the odds of pregnancy achievement, are thoroughly discussed in *Taking Charge of Your Fertility.*

❋ THE BIRDS AND BEES IN APPROPRIATE CONTEXT

Despite my strong belief that FAM should not be used by teenage girls, I am well aware that a book about observing fertility signs and charting cycles has certain contraceptive implications, and regardless, is logically intertwined with a host of issues related to sexuality. Since the primary aim of this book is to empower my readers with the necessary knowledge to take charge of their cycles and gynecological health, I deal with those tangential sexual issues—from birth control to sexually transmitted infections (STIs)—in a way that I believe is both responsible and consistent with that goal.

This is to say that I do think there are many valid reasons why teens should abstain from sexual activity, and those reasons are, in fact, discussed later in the appropriate context. However, this book cannot take an "abstinence only" approach to fertility education, because it is simply unrealistic to think that most girls will remain abstinent just because they are encouraged to do so. I believe that they are more likely to postpone intercourse, though, if they develop a profound respect for their bodies that comes with the knowledge gained from charting their cycles. As a women's health educator, I believe in presenting all relevant and appropriate information that will help keep my readers both healthy and safe.

Ultimately, though, this book is no more a sex-education manual than it is a primer on tampons. It is about your daughter's remarkable body, and the signs she'll need to learn in order to understand what it is telling her, from puberty to menopause. Still, a book can't replace years of experience, and thus I would hope that you will always be there to answer her questions and address her concerns.

If you yourself have yet to learn the basic principles of Fertility Awareness, I encourage you to read this book as well. You'll then be able to intelligently discuss virtually any menstrual issue, which is a good thing in itself. For if your daughter feels comfortable confiding in you about her cervical fluid, for example, she'll certainly be a lot more likely to discuss other personal issues—menstrual, sexual, or otherwise! So may you both learn from each other, but most importantly, it is my sincere hope that your daughter will soon be biologically self-aware in the truest sense of those words—a powerful foundation as she steadily matures into a confident young woman.

introduction

SHE SAID *WHAT*?

i'll never forget the surprising comment my mom made that sunny afternoon when I was about 15 years old. It had been one of those days when it seemed like nothing had gone right, and I was feeling pretty down. To top it off, I had my period and was feeling crampy and hardly the picture of joy and harmony. So what did I do? I did what any self-respecting teenager would do in a situation like that: I started complaining to my mom about periods and how stupid they were.

I mean, there you are, living your life, when all of a sudden, blood just starts flowing between your legs. How weird is that? And it's not enough that it happens once in a while. No, it happens about once a month, from the time you start menstruating until you go through menopause some 40 years later. Helloooooo? Who came up with *that* idea?

But leave it to my mom to respond in a way that left me scratching my head. She said that she had never minded periods, because they made her feel feminine. Excuse me? Yes, feminine! She said that about once a month, she was reminded that her body was so amazing and unique, and so different from a man's, that she actually celebrated it during that week or so.

OK, now don't get me wrong. My initial reaction was probably similar to yours. Celebrate bleeding once a month? I don't *think* so. But the funny thing is, ever since that fateful day, I started carrying myself just a little differently during my period. Even feeling a little more confident. My body was pretty cool, and capable of doing things that my three brothers' bodies would never do!

And you know what I realized years later? My mom was actually onto something. It turns out that in many cultures throughout the world, menstruation isn't considered an illness, a curse, or even a nuisance. It's a positive sign of health. In many societies, it's a time of celebration. A rite of passage.

So snuggle up in a comfy chair and start learning how to view your entire menstrual cycle as not only as a source of self-revelation, but also of feminine pride and pure biological wonder.

part one

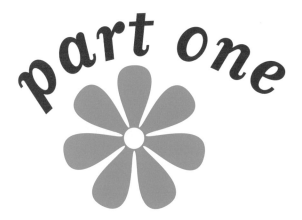

CYCLE
SMART

those hip, happenin' hormones

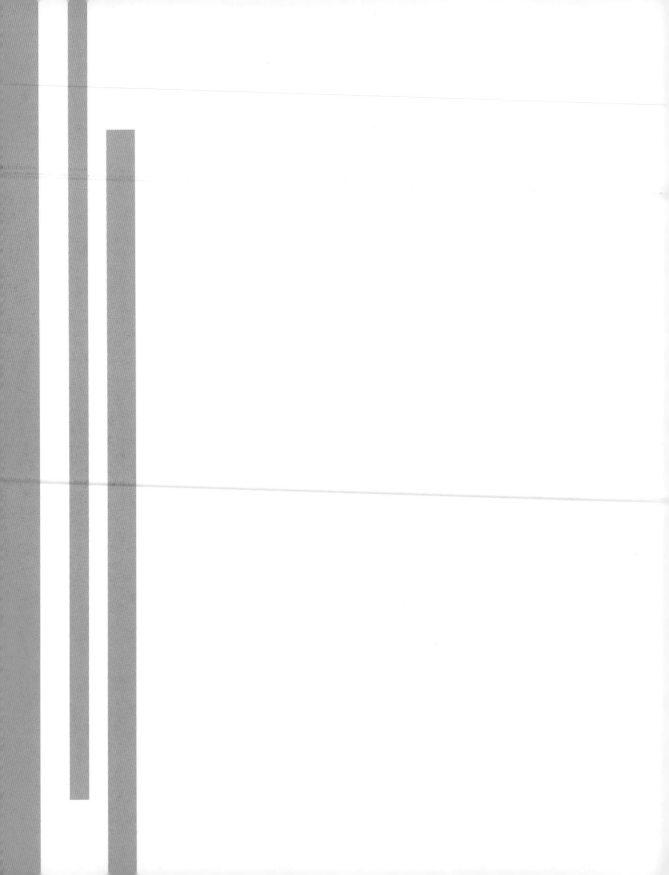

one

YOUR AMAZING
AND AWESOME BODY

do you realize that you actually started your life inside your *grandmother*? Huh? How is that possible? Well, the very egg that eventually became you was originally inside your mother's ovaries when she was but a fetus inside her own pregnant mother! Another way of saying this is that every woman who is pregnant with a female fetus is carrying a part of her potential grandchildren in her body. What? Keep reading.

Let's go back to when your mom was just a fetus. Female fetuses already contain all the eggs that they will ever have. Practically speaking, that means that when your mother was a fetus inside *her* mother, she had already developed one of the eggs that eventually became you. So if she was 35 years old when she had you, and you are now 16, the cells inside of you today that were once part of the egg that became you would be about 51! The best way to help you grasp this fascinating concept is to simply fill in the lines next to the illustration on the following page with the appropriate names.

3

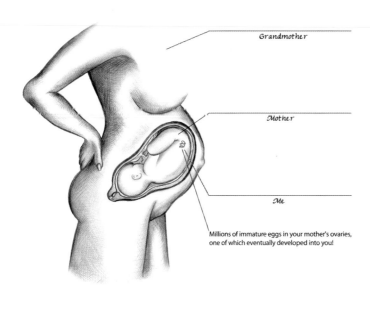

Grandmother

Mother

Me

Millions of immature eggs in your mother's ovaries, one of which eventually developed into you!

One of the major differences between male and female anatomy has to do with when the sex cells (or gametes) are developed. As you just read, girls are born with all the eggs they will ever have. Yet the eggs don't mature until puberty, when about one egg per cycle is released. This continues all the way through menopause (the time when a woman stops having periods altogether). Boys, on the other hand, don't develop sperm until adolescence, but then continually produce sperm every day until they die.

✱ YOUR EXTERNAL REPRODUCTIVE ANATOMY

If you have a brother close in age to you, you may remember taking baths with him as a toddler and being perplexed as to why he had this "thing" on the outside that you didn't have. He might have even gleefully pointed down there while boasting about it. Even from a very young age, boys in our society are usually socialized to believe they possess a treasure in which to take pride, whereas girls tend to grow up embarrassed about what they have "down there." Well, that's got to change, here and now.

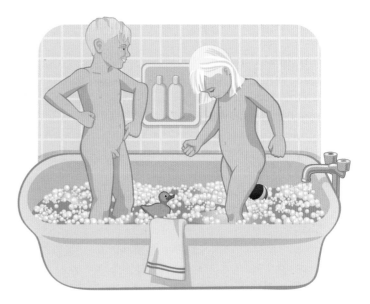

As you know, you have a vagina while boys have a penis. No big surprise there. But what you probably didn't know is that, in terms of pleasure, your vagina is actually not the female counterpart of his penis—your *clitoris* is (my *what* is?).

As you'll see, your clitoris (pronounced kli-'tor-əs) is *your* "special thing." So even though your vagina is one of the things that makes you a girl, your clitoris makes being a girl, well, more fun! There will be more on this a bit later (in Chapter 6), but for now, it's back to your vagina, which should be a healthy pink color, like the inside of your cheek. It has three distinct functions: It's a passageway for the flow of menstrual blood, a flexible muscle that surrounds a penis when a woman has intercourse with a man, and a birth canal for an emerging baby during childbirth.

What protects your vagina are your *vaginal lips*. They vary in size, shape, and color. Books always refer to two sets—the inner lips, or labia minora, and the outer lips, or labia majora. But in reality, the only ones that are truly protective and even remotely resemble lips are the inner ones. The outer lips are really not lips at all, but more of a soft hair-covered padding.

> *The first time I caught a glimpse of vaginal lips was when I was maybe three or four years old. I remember squatting on the floor in the bathroom while my mom peed, and being completely confused by what I saw between her legs as she stood up from the toilet. From that angle, they looked really strange.*
>
> —Brie, 19

You can imagine how a toddler might find many things in her young life confusing or frightening if she has never seen them before. Luckily, as children get older, things that were once scary can often become really intriguing and beautiful with familiarity. So it is with vaginal lips.

Now, you wouldn't wear a dress to the prom without viewing it from every angle, would you? Yet, in a certain way, you wear your external anatomy every day. Aren't you just a tad curious? The only way you are going to know what I've been talking about these last few pages is if you actually look down there yourself! I realize that sounds pretty extreme, maybe even a little intimidating, but consider this: a boy sees and touches his penis every time he goes to the bathroom. Perhaps that's why boys seem more comfortable with their bodies and sexuality. Why can't you, a girl, feel the same? Now you can!

You can build respect for your body by becoming more familiar with all its important parts, including those below your belly. So read the next three pages, then find a private place, and grab that mirror. It's time you get to know your own body as well as boys know theirs!

Exploring Down There

TAKE OUT THAT MIRROR AND GET TO KNOW YOURSELF

Find some time after a shower or bath when you are clean, have complete privacy and enough time to relax, and explore what makes you, you. Did you know that the external appearance of your sexual anatomy is as unique as your face? It's true. So the sooner you become familiar with your body, the easier it will be for you to develop a real sense of wonder about it.

Use whatever type of mirror is most comfortable: a handheld or even a wall mirror, as long as it allows you to see yourself in bright light while you are seated in a comfortable position, legs open and bent at the knees.

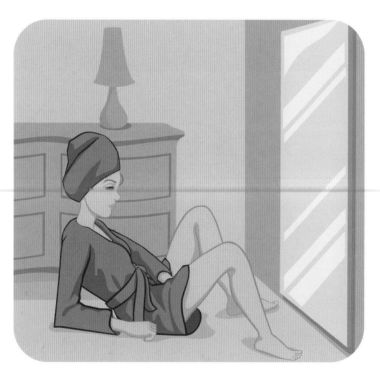

Familiarize yourself with your **vulva,** which is the term used to describe the entire external part of your anatomy between your legs. Notice the difference between your soft, hair-covered mound **(labia majora)** and your actual vaginal lips **(labia minora).** Notice whether your lips are pink or brown, thin or protruding, smooth or wrinkled. All of these variations are normal.

Just above the point where your vaginal lips meet at the top, you will find a pea-shaped bulge that is filled with sexual nerves. What you actually see is the tip of your **clitoris**, but the entire structure extends much farther inside your body as well. It is your clitoris, and not your vagina, that is the center of most sexual pleasure.

With clean hands, spread your vaginal lips to reveal two distinct openings. The tiny opening near the top is your **urethra**, the narrow tube that carries urine out of your body.

The larger opening just below that is your **vagina**. It is the elastic muscular passageway to your uterus. Just inside your vagina, you may find a thin protective membrane of skin called a **hymen**. Not all girls are born with one, and many girls naturally stretch it out in the course of regular activities such as exercise or even inserting tampons. If it is still in place at the time of first intercourse, it will usually be stretched open then.

Your vagina is usually pink and moist. You'll notice that its walls remain touching unless you manually separate them. Your vaginal walls are comprised of hundreds of tiny folds that allow it to stretch and accommodate whatever is inside, such as a tampon, a penis, or even a baby! One of the easiest ways to see how muscular it can be is to insert a finger inside and squeeze all around your finger. Do you see how much control you have over your vagina?

The last thing you can feel while exploring your vulva is actually farther up inside at the end of your vagina. It is your **cervix**, the opening of your uterus. If you insert your clean middle finger as far as it will go, you will find it. It will probably feel similar to the firmness of the tip of your nose or the softness of your lips, depending on what point you are in your cycle. You'll notice that right in the middle of it is a tiny opening, called the **os**. It is through this opening that your menstrual blood flows from your uterus, and more remarkably, where a baby will one day pass through if you ever give birth.

I was so excited to start shaving my legs. Not that there was much to shave but some light, soft hair. But it proved that I was growing up and was no longer a child. One day I was horrified to discover one dark pubic hair. The only hair that I had ever seen like that was a man's beard. I thought something was really wrong with me. I quickly grabbed my razor and shaved it off! Of course it grew back with lots more. By this time I knew this was normal for women.

—Jane, 14

WHAT MAKES YOU A GIRL ON THE OUTSIDE

Vulva The external female genitals.

Mons pubis The soft fleshy tissue beneath the pubic hair that protects the internal reproductive organs.

Hood of clitoris The protective covering of the clitoris, formed by the joining of the two inner vaginal lips.

Clitoris The pea-sized organ that becomes filled with blood during sexual arousal, causing it to become firm and erect. As the primary site of orgasm for the majority of women, it is filled with more sexual nerve endings than any other part of the body. It is the female counterpart to the tip of the male penis.

Outer vaginal lips (labia majora) Soft padding, which contains oil-producing glands and a small amount of pubic hair.

Inner vaginal lips (labia minora) Folds of very soft, sleek skin. Typically covers the vagina unless the woman becomes sexually aroused, at which point the inner lips tend to fill with blood and blossom out. They may also become full and separate around ovulation.

Urethra The narrow tube that carries urine from the bladder out of the body.

Vaginal opening (introitus) The outer entrance to the vagina. The opening for the release of menstrual blood as well as cervical fluid. The site through which a baby's head emerges during childbirth.

Vagina The elastic 4- to 6-inch-long muscular passage between the vulva and cervix that acts as the passageway for the flow of menstrual blood, the receptor of the penis during intercourse, and the birth canal during childbirth.

Anus The opening at the end of the digestive tract.

Bartholin's glands Two tiny glands, one on each side of the vaginal opening, that produce a thin lubricant when a woman becomes sexually aroused.

Perineum The membrane between the vaginal opening and the anus that remarkably stretches during childbirth to allow a baby's head to pass through the vaginal opening.

❋ YOUR INTERNAL REPRODUCTIVE ANATOMY

Alas, exploring your internal reproductive organs is a little more challenging, unless you happen to own an X-ray machine for an occasional glimpse inside. Needless to say, the star of your reproductive system is your uterus, or womb, but in many ways, your ovaries play an even more important role in the actual process of reproduction. The main purpose of your uterus is to provide a cozy place in which a fetus can develop into a baby. And even though you probably won't have a baby for years, if ever, your body prepares for that possibility every single menstrual cycle by building up the lining of your uterus, and shedding it if a pregnancy does not occur. What allows this event to happen every month or so is the hormonal drama that continually evolves in the amazing little powerhouses of your ovaries, all of which will be discussed in the next chapter.

Before moving on, you'll want to get a better feel for your inner anatomy and its functions (really, so don't skip this!). Even though the illustration below won't allow you to experience that up-close-and-personal exploration of your body the way you could with your outer vulva, it should still give you a clear idea of the purpose of your inner organs.

WHAT MAKES YOU A GIRL ON THE INSIDE

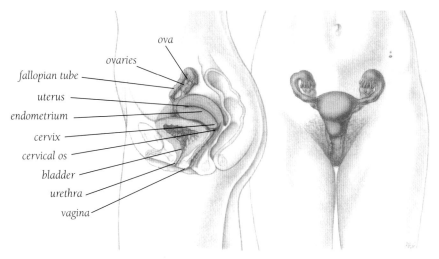

Is there anything on the left side of this illustration that surprises you? Many girls are surprised to discover that, for most women, the natural position of the uterus is tipped forward. Also, do you notice how the uterus sits just above the bladder where urine is stored? Now maybe you can understand why your mom probably had to run to the bathroom every other minute when she was pregnant with you!

CROSS-SECTION OF UTERUS

Uterus The womb. A hollow, muscular, pear-shaped organ (about the size of a small lemon) that builds up and releases a blood-rich lining every cycle and acts as an "incubator" for the developing fetus if conception occurs. In most women, the uterus curves forward.

Fallopian tubes The 4- to 5-inch-long narrow tubes through which the egg travels from the ovary to the uterus, and where conception takes place.

Ova (singular: ovum) Granule-sized eggs stored in the ovaries, one of which is usually released each cycle. An ovulated ovum may unite with a sperm in one of the fallopian tubes to form the fertilized egg that eventually becomes a fetus.

Ovaries Two almond-sized primary sex glands that contain at least a million immature eggs at birth. Each egg (or ovum) is surrounded by a group of cells called a follicle. The ovaries produce the hormones estrogen and progesterone throughout the reproductive years.

Endometrium The lining of the uterus, which builds up in preparation for a potential pregnancy and is shed every cycle in the form of menstruation if conception and implantation did not occur.

Cervix The lower opening of the uterus. The only part of the uterus that can be felt protruding into the upper vagina. Lined with channels that cyclically develop cervical fluid in which sperm can thrive up to a week.

Cervical os The small opening of the cervix that dilates around ovulation and expands to allow a baby to pass through during childbirth.

Vagina The elastic 4- to 6-inch-long muscular passage between the vulva and cervix that acts as the passageway for the flow of menstrual blood. During sexual arousal and intercourse, the vagina expands to accommodate a penis, and it stretches during childbirth to accommodate a baby.

❋ APPLES AND ORANGES, BOYS AND GIRLS

Do you remember how this chapter started? You filled in your name and the names of your mom and grandmother, right? That's because I wanted you to appreciate the magic of reproduction and understand the concept that girls are born with all the eggs they will ever have. But it's very different for boys.

The box below reflects the three major differences between male and female fertility, which is technically the word that's used to indicate the ability to make a baby. As you will see, boys become fertile when they start making sperm at puberty (usually around the time their voices start changing). Girls become fertile when they start having menstrual cycles at puberty, and finally begin releasing the eggs they were born with.

DIFFERENCES BETWEEN FEMALE AND MALE FERTILITY

Women	Men
Fertile only a few days per cycle, since the release of an egg (ovulation) occurs only once per cycle	Fertile all the time, since sperm are produced on a daily basis
Fertile from puberty until menopause (which occurs at about 50 years old)	Fertile from puberty until death
Born with all the eggs they will ever have, but don't start to release them until puberty	Not born with any sperm, but start to produce them at puberty

Of course, eggs don't just start popping out willy-nilly. In the next chapter, you'll learn about the hormonal drama that occurs each month in your almond-shaped ovaries, the place where your eggs hang out until their potential release each and every cycle. And what a drama it is!

Are you cycle logical?

See How Well You Understood Chapter 1

Answer the questions on pages 13 and 14. Then record them down the columns of this puzzle to discover the hidden phrase in the bold outline.
Answers on page 176, but no peeking.

1	2	3	4	5		6	7	8	9	10

1. Vaginal lips vary from woman to woman in size, shape, and _____.
   color
   location
   function

2. If a woman experiences this, she will not get her period the next cycle:
   a vaginal infection
   a bad hair day
   pregnancy

3. This is filled with more sexual nerves than anywhere else on the female body:
   vagina
   clitoris
   belly button

4. What your finger should be before you feel your cervix:
   manicured
   clean
   long

5. Unlike men, who are fertile from puberty until they die, women are only fertile from puberty until _____, the time in their life when they stop having periods.
   menopause
   their late 30s
   they're fed up with having periods

6. Girl babies are born with about a million immature ones of these in their ovaries:
   children
   cells
   eggs

7. One of two internal tubes in which the egg is fertilized:
   test tube
   endometrial tube
   fallopian tube

8. A muscular passage between the vulva and the cervix. (Between the what and the where? I told you to get out that mirror!)

    vagina

    cervical os

    clitoris

9. The name of the opening of the uterus (it's got an opening?):

    navel

    cervix

    fallopian tube

10. The protective membrane of skin just inside the vagina that may be naturally stretched out during regular activities or at the time of first intercourse:

    hymen

    lowmen

    foreskin

two

WHO KNEW?

The Fun Between Your Periods

*h*ave you ever thought about how different life would be if boys got periods rather than girls? Like you, I suspect many would be nervous while waiting for their first one. Unlike you, though, once they had experienced a couple of them and the fear had passed, a lot of those guys would probably figure out a way to brag among themselves about just how much blood they'd lost ("Hey, dude, I bet I bleed more than you." "No way, maaan. I lost, like, two cups this morning!"). Hmmm, ya gotta love boys, right?

In reality, of course, periods are often seen as a critical part of what it means to be female, and you might have been filled with anticipation just waiting for the first one to arrive in the year or so before it did. And yet, no matter how routine your period has now become in your life, when you think about it, there really is something pretty weird about bleeding, cycle after cycle after cycle.

Throw in the physical hassles that are often part of the whole experience, from tampons and pads to cramps and bad-bathing-suit days, and it's understandable why most women think that menstrual periods are the central event of every cycle. But in truth, something far less obvious is the main event. Keep reading, and you'll soon discover what it is!

> *The day I got my period was the most confusing day of my life. I was only 10 and I was in science class when I felt like I had just peed a bit in my underwear. My teacher wouldn't let me go to the bathroom, and hours later when I was finally allowed to go I couldn't figure out what this red spot was on my underwear. I thought I was bleeding and I put layers of toilet paper in my underwear. After a few more hours of discomfort I got home and my mom explained to me what was going on. I hated it. I cried for hours.*
>
> —*Larissa, 15*

What would have made Larissa's experience exciting rather than confusing? Knowledge. If only she had known what to expect, she could have looked forward to her period as a new stage in her life. Still, while it's true that periods are the most noticeable part of your cycle, the more you learn about how your body works and why it does what it does, the faster you'll realize that at least in terms of basic female biology, periods are really no big deal. In fact, in some ways their most important function is simply to let you know when one cycle has ended and another has begun. Of course, that doesn't tell you anything about why we even have cycles to begin with.

It's in answering this question of why that you'll soon learn something truly fundamental about yourself: While so many of your worries and emotions are often centered on menstruation, your body is actually focused on *ovulation*. That's because in reality, ovulation is the central event of your cycle, not menstruation, as most people think.

OK, that sounds intriguing, but what does ovulation really mean? Well, technically, it is simply the release of an egg from your ovary. Sounds like a real snoozer compared to the fun of cramps, blood, tampons, and Midol, right? Yet to really understand why ovulation is so critical, you need to know this most basic biological fact: *Your body prepares for a potential pregnancy, each and every cycle.* And that's something worth really understanding!

Yep, once you've started menstruating, you are very likely ovulating, and that means you are physically capable of getting pregnant, no matter how young you are when you get your first period.

> *I knew absolutely NOTHING about fertility and my mother sure didn't tell me anything. When I got my period, I told my mother and her only response was "Well, you know you can get pregnant now." I was, like— I can? Talk about a non-existent sex talk!*
>
> *—Kendra, 18*

It's a pretty intense thing to realize that once you start having periods, you can get pregnant. That alone should convince you why it's so important to learn just how your menstrual cycle works. Sure, you could just think of it as "female biology" (yawn), but over the next few pages, let's step back and learn about something far more interesting: You.

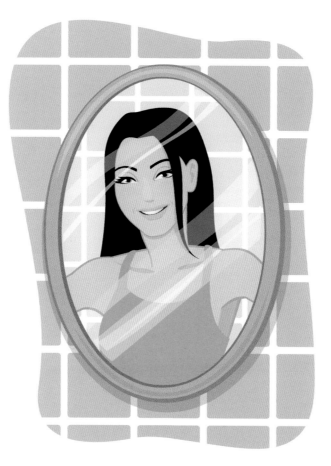

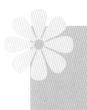

Menstrual Fun Facts

Menstruation	The cyclical shedding of the uterine lining
Menses (MEN-zeez)	Another word for menstruation
Menarche (MEN-are-kee)	The age at which menstruation begins. For American girls, the average age is 12, but most girls begin menstruating between 10 and 14. In fact, it's generally believed that girls today are getting their periods at a younger age than a few generations ago, although the reasons for this are not clear.
Menstrual cycle	From the first day of bleeding to the day before the next bleeding
Average length of a menstrual cycle	About 28 days
Normal menstrual cycle length variation	24 to 36 days
Average length of a period	5 days
Average amount of blood lost during each period	Only about 4 tablespoons (surprising, huh?)
What menstrual blood comprises	A combination of blood, mucus, and pieces of the uterine lining (clots). Prior to flowing out of a woman's body, menstrual blood was the uterine lining that developed to provide nourishment and protection for a potential fetus.
The four factors that can best support a healthy menstrual cycle	A good diet, plenty of exercise, enough sleep, and sleeping in a dark room
The one question you never want to take too literally	May I borrow a tampon?

❋ THOSE CLEVER HORMONES INSIDE YOU

Hormones. You've probably heard of them numerous times, but what the heck are they, and how do they work? Everyone has them, male and female, and they affect many different physical functions. While one can spend years studying hormones in great detail, the most important thing to know at this point is simply that they are powerful, natural chemicals produced in one organ of the body that are carried to other parts of the body through the bloodstream.

Although hormones were not a noticeable part of your life when you were a kid, their later appearance is what led you into puberty. You may have already heard that your cycles are largely controlled by a group of several distinct hormones. But before you dismiss them as totally borrrrring, consider this: It's the emergence of four key reproductive hormones that is responsible for most of the physical changes you've been going through over these last few years. That includes everything from the cool and interesting (growing breasts, curvier hips, and fluffy pubic hair) to the not-so-cool and yucky (menstrual cramps, mood swings, and zits). So yeah, hormones matter a lot, and if you aren't at least a bit familiar with the most important ones, you can't really understand yourself, much less your cycles!

> *When I was younger, my breasts developed before any other girl in my class. It was more fat than anything else, but I was still embarrassed by them. I had to start wearing bras in the third or fourth grade and I always told my mom that the bras fit when really they were three sizes too small for me. I wanted my breasts compressed. Sometimes I even layered tight bras or put an Ace bandage around myself to flatten them more. I was so embarrassed about my body that I caused myself a lot of pain.*
>
> *—Olivia, 15*

Does Olivia's story above sound familiar? Girls all develop at different times, so it's understandable that sometimes you might feel a little self-conscious if you grow at a faster pace than others in your grade.

But back to the hormones that lead to all these changes in your body. Three of them appear in your body in the first part of your cycle, leading up to ovulation. They are called, in order of appearance, follicle-stimulating hormone (FSH), estrogen, and luteinizing hormone (LH). The last hormone, progesterone, appears in your body after you've ovulated. As mentioned earlier, ovulation is the most important event in every cycle, so you should also know its place in the general order of the hormones.

All of this will be easy to learn if you just memorize the acronym FELOP (which, of course, stands for Fawns Eat Lots of Pickles):

>**F**ollicle-stimulating hormone
>**E**strogen
>**L**uteinizing hormone
>**O**VULATION
>**P**rogesterone

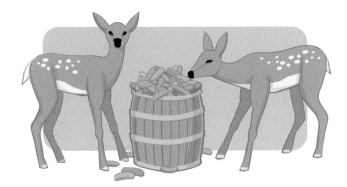

You may have noticed I wrote that the first three hormones appear in the first part of your cycle, before ovulation, but I didn't say the first *half*. That's because while ovulation can and often does occur at about the halfway point of any cycle, it certainly doesn't have to. In fact, when it occurs varies among women as well as within individual women.

More specifically, and despite what you may have heard (drum roll, please):

NOT ALL CYCLES ARE 28 DAYS, AND OVULATION DOES NOT ALWAYS OCCUR ON DAY 14!

In fact, it's quite common for cycles to be considerably longer, and for reasons that you'll soon understand, it's also common for ovulation to occur closer to the end of the cycle than the beginning. This is especially true for teenagers such as yourself.

There is a simple but important fact as to why this is true: The amount of time from the first day of your period to the day you ovulate can vary quite a bit, while the amount of time from ovulation to your next cycle remains remarkably consistent, usually never varying for any individual by more than a day or two. Unfortunately, most people (including many doctors!) do not realize that the preovulatory phase of the cycle often takes from as few as 10 or 11 days to as many as 20 days or longer. (Are your eyes glazing over yet? Give them a good rub and keep reading—it will all become crystal clear very soon.) I'll explain why that is, and why the postovulatory phase is so regular. For now, though, it's enough to understand that while ovulation can take place on Day 14 of your cycle, it can also occur sooner or considerably later.

Don't Fall into the 28-Day Cycle Trap!

When I was younger, every time I got my period, I thought of it as either two days early, if it was a 26-day cycle, or three days late, if it was a 31-day cycle, or four days early, if it was . . . well, you get the idea. I maintained this kind of thinking for years and years until my late 20s. Why? Because like you, most of us grow up hearing that a 28-day cycle is the norm.

But where does that myth come from? Part of it has to do with what I call the pill mentality. One of the reasons for the 28-day belief is the popularity of the contraceptive pill, which is designed to produce a perfect 28-day cycle. Because so many women use the Pill, they have come to believe that a normal menstrual cycle is always 28 days. The one little detail that is missing from the big picture, though, is that the Pill *artificially* manipulates your cycle!

In reality, women are not robots. Nor are we Barbie dolls. So we shouldn't expect that our bodies will all be alike and work like clockwork every single cycle. So, while it's true that many of you will have natural 28-day cycles, you should know that normal cycles range from about 24 to 36 days.

There are several unfortunate consequences of the Pill Mentality. One is that people's idea of what is considered a normal cycle becomes distorted. Another is that while on the Pill, you don't ovulate, so you miss out on the opportunity to be totally in tune with your female patterns. Remember that before and after ovulation, your cycles naturally ebb and flow (no pun intended . . . well, OK, maybe a little bit intended), which is a pretty cool thing, when you think about it. But on the Pill, you miss out on all of that. And finally, the pill mentality encourages women to simply accept numerous side effects and physical risks in exchange for contraceptive convenience.

❋ DETAILS, DETAILS: THE BIOLOGY OF MENSTRUATION

I can hear the groans already: "Biology? Snooooze." But trust me—you're not going to want to skip this! The beauty of your body is in its details. It's time to step back and see what your body is really up to as you progress through every cycle. As you continue reading, keep in mind that menstruation is more than just "that time of the month." It's a positive sign of health. Remember, in many cultures, it's a time of celebration. A rite of passage. Hey, it's a powerful symbol of being female, even of femininity itself!

Let's start with Day 1, which is the first day of menstruation. As you've learned, however, it is not the most important day; that title belongs to the day of ovulation.

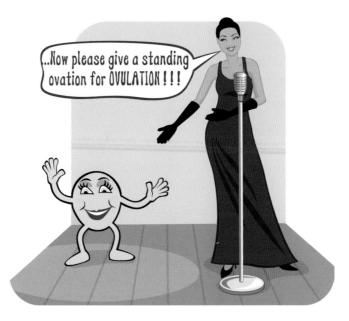

When your period starts, a new cycle begins, but it's important to understand that menstruation is a direct result of the events of your previous cycle—just as colorful autumn leaves arise from the full green trees of summer. So while we consider menstruation the beginning of a new cycle, the truth is that bleeding marks the end of the cycle before. Regardless, the reason we still consider the beginning of your period as Day 1 is that it would be much trickier to identify the exact day you ovulate as the first day of your cycle!

In any case, why the bleeding, and why now? The weeks before you began to menstruate, the wall of your uterus, or endometrium, became thick with blood and nutrients, and thus reached the goal necessary for its only purpose: to provide the appropriate conditions to nurture a fertilized egg (often called an embryo) if you had become pregnant that cycle.

> *I remember the day I started to have my first really heavy period. I was extremely embarrassed and didn't ask my mom or older sister if I could use a pad. Instead, I went to school using a wad of rolled-up toilet paper. Unfortunately, the toilet paper was insufficient and caused me to leak through my pants. The stain on my pants was pointed out to me near the end of the school day by a friend, and since then, I've always felt the need to wear dark pants and a sweatshirt around my waist when menstruating. Fortunately, with time and experience, the need for extra security faded away.*
>
> *—Betsy, 19*

What causes you to start bleeding is a sudden plunge in your progesterone (for reasons to be explained later), the hormone that had kept the uterine wall nourished and in place. Now, on Day 1, with no progesterone left to maintain it, the lining of the uterus gradually dissolves and begins to flow through the cervix and out your vagina. For you, of course, all of this is your period, usually lasting about five or six days. Congratulations! The dramatic menstrual events that mark the first phase of your reproductive cycle have officially begun.

❋ THE ROAD TO OVULATION

It is worth noting here that as your period begins, none of the key "FELOP" hormones are present in significant quantity (remember, Fawns Eat Lots Of Pickles). However, as you continue menstruating, the first of these hormones, follicle-stimulating hormone (FSH), starts to increase in your body. During the first couple weeks of every cycle, FSH is responsible for the development of about 15 to 20 eggs, which start to grow bigger in each of your two ovaries. Each egg is encased in a protective covering of cells called a follicle—hence how FSH, or follicle-stimulating hormone, got its name. These maturing cells begin to produce increasing amounts of estrogen, the second of your key FELOP hormones.

Starting about the second week of most cycles, an exciting race develops in your otherwise peaceful ovaries. It is now a contest between those rapidly maturing follicles, in which each one is trying to become the largest and most dominant. This is an event worth participating in, since the winning egg eventually breaks out of its casing and right through the walls of your ovary! But before that can happen, one more key development is necessary to propel all the contestants toward the finish line.

As the follicles release more and more estrogen into your body, a signal is eventually sent to your brain to begin producing one last chemical, called luteinizing hormone (LH). LH plays a critical role in helping those competing eggs to continue maturing, but it is best known for a sudden surge that brings this contest to a close. Biologists refer to this as the LH surge, and it is this hormonal phenomenon that thrusts the winning egg right through the ovarian wall. (At this point, the other developing eggs in the ovary basically disintegrate. Sad, but true.) Finally, the victorious egg tumbles into the pelvic cavity, where it is quickly swept into one of the fallopian tubes.

These dramatic events, which you now know as ovulation, mark the end of your cycle's preovulatory phase and the beginning of its postovulatory phase. For most of your life, that one special egg every cycle will not be fertilized, but if you one day have children, conception will have occurred in your fallopian tubes, from where the fertilized egg will begin the long journey all the way down to your uterus.

Cool Facts About Ovulation

- The race to release an egg can take anywhere from about 10 to 20 days or even longer to complete, although it averages about two weeks.

- In the days leading up to ovulation, you will experience various primary fertility signs, including progressively wetter secretions that you will probably notice on your underwear. These secretions, called cervical fluid, are perfectly normal, and are discussed in the next chapter.

- You may even experience a day or two of red, pink, or brown blood right around ovulation, often referred to as ovulatory spotting.

- You can only ovulate once per cycle. However, within a single ovulation, and more specifically, within 24 hours of that first egg bursting through its ovarian wall, a second egg will occasionally sneak out. This is called multiple ovulation. If both eggs are fertilized, this is what causes fraternal twins, the type of twins who develop from two different eggs and who don't necessarily look any more alike than typical siblings do.

- Assuming only one egg is released during a particular ovulation, it is random as to which ovary ultimately releases the egg. Ovulation doesn't necessarily alternate between ovaries, as is often thought.

- Around ovulation, you may feel a sharp or dull pain in your lower abdomen that lasts from a few minutes to a few hours. It is usually referred to as ovulatory pain.

- It is possible for a girl to get pregnant even if she has not started menstruating yet, because ovulation always occurs about two weeks *before* menstruation.

Before we move on from ovulation, however, it is important to repeat that the first, or preovulatory, part of the cycle—from Day 1 of your period until you ovulate—can vary considerably in length (the preovulatory phase is sometimes called the follicular phase, because the follicles in your ovary are developing). On the other hand, the second or postovulatory phase of your cycle—from ovulation to your next period—usually has a finite life span of 12 to 16 days. This means that *it is the day of ovulation that determines the total length of your cycle,* and more importantly for you, when you can expect the first day of your next period.

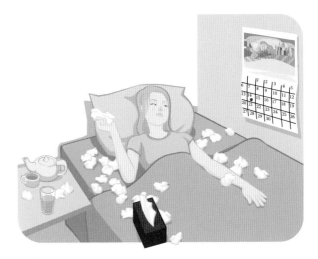

For instance, you could have an extremely delayed ovulation for all kinds of reasons, from a nasty flu that wipes you out for a few weeks to stress over a huge homework assignment. If this were to happen, you might not ovulate, for example, until about Day 30 of that cycle. That means you could end up with a 44-day cycle (30 preovulatory days plus approximately 14 postovulatory days). So just because a woman hasn't gotten her period by Day 44, it doesn't necessarily mean that she's pregnant!

❋ FROM OVULATION TO THE END OF YOUR CYCLE

After the release of the egg from the ovary, the follicular casing that held the egg collapses, becoming a corpus luteum, or literally, a "yellow body." It remains essentially stuck on the interior ovarian wall, where it immediately starts releasing progesterone (the last of the key FELOP hormones, and yes, it's still true that Fawns Eat Lots of Pickles). It is important to note that the corpus luteum has a set life span of about 12 to 16 days, rarely varying by more than a couple of days within each individual woman. (Because the corpus luteum produces the hormones for the postovulatory phase, it is often called the "luteal phase.")

So if your best friend Sophie's postovulatory phase is normally 13 days, for example, it may occasionally be 12 days and occasionally 14, but it is rarely outside that range. This is because the corpus luteum is unaffected by horrible colds, overdue homework, outrageous boyfriends, and all the other stresses of everyday life. The corpus luteum will produce progesterone no matter what else is going on in your life. So stress, both physical and emotional, can impact the number of days before you ovulate, but rarely the number of days after ovulation (phew). Got it? Good.

Progesterone is important in a woman's cycle, and more specifically, for a woman's fertility, because it does three things:

1. Prevents the release of all other eggs for that cycle.
2. Causes the uterine lining (endometrium) to thicken and maintain itself until the corpus luteum disintegrates, 12 to 16 days later.
3. Causes the two primary fertility signs to change (these signs are waking temperature and cervical fluid, both discussed in the next chapter).

In a small percentage of cycles, two or more eggs are released during ovulation, but always within a 24-hour period. As you've read, this phenomenon is called "multiple ovulation," and is responsible for fraternal twins. (Identical twins develop from one single egg that splits in two, so, of course, they look like the name implies: identical!)

More eggs cannot be released later that cycle (beyond that 24-hour period) due to the powerful effects of progesterone mentioned above. Progesterone quickly stops the release of all other eggs until the next cycle, and if a woman does become pregnant, it stops the release of any more eggs for the duration of that pregnancy. So a woman cannot release an egg one day, get pregnant, and then release an egg again weeks or months later! Basically, her body protects that potential pregnancy by preventing her from being able to release more eggs following that ovulation. If she could, she'd be having a baby every few weeks, undoubtedly landing her on the cover of her favorite supermarket tabloid!

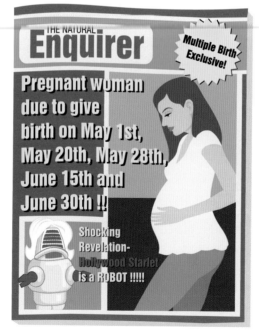

Once the egg bursts through the ovarian wall, it actually floats briefly in your abdominal cavity before it gets swept into the fallopian tube by the fimbria, which are the tube's fingerlike tendrils. Assuming it is not fertilized by a sperm, the egg remains alive for a maximum of 24 hours. After that, it simply dissolves and either is reabsorbed by the body or comes out in the menstrual flow. However, since the egg is about the size of the dot in the exclamation point at the end of this sentence, it's not likely that you would ever notice it hanging out on a maxi pad!

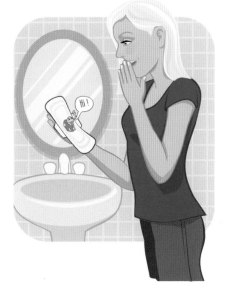

Finally, you should be aware that you might occasionally not release an egg at all. This is referred to as an "anovulatory cycle." These cycles may range from very short to extremely long, and are further discussed in the box on the following two pages.

Three boys are sitting on the stoop one summer afternoon. One of their fathers, exasperated that the kids are just sitting around, gives them five bucks and tells them to go amuse themselves. As they walk down Main Street, they debate what they should do with the money. Should they buy a deck of cards? A football? Play in the arcade?

"Wait a sec!" says one of the boys as he runs into the drugstore. "Wait here!"

A few minutes later he comes out with a package of tampons.

"You idiot!" his friends shout. "We were going to have some fun. What are we going to do with those?"

"Look what it says right here on the box," the boy replies: "'You can go horseback riding, you can go swimming, you can...'"

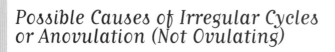

Possible Causes of Irregular Cycles or Anovulation (Not Ovulating)

BEING A TEENAGER!

When girls first start menstruating and even throughout their teen years, their cycles may be irregular as their body adjusts to releasing an egg every cycle.

ILLNESS

Being sick does not necessarily affect your cycle, but if it does, it usually either delays ovulation or prevents it altogether, assuming you get sick *before* you ovulate. Remember, the postovulatory phase is fairly consistent and usually unaffected by external events.

STRESS

One of the most likely causes of occasional long cycles is stress, either physiological or psychological. If stress affects a cycle at all, it tends to delay ovulation, not hasten it. The timing of ovulation will determine the length of the cycle—the later it occurs, the longer the cycle will be. Sometimes, if stress is severe, it can prevent ovulation altogether.

TRAVEL

Traveling is notorious for affecting cycles, often by delaying ovulation and lengthening the cycle. Some women even stop ovulating and getting periods until they quit traveling.

HEAVY EXERCISE

Strenuous exercise has the potential to delay or even prevent ovulation. Although you may be tempted to use this as an excuse not to exercise, don't! It seems to affect mostly those who are competitive athletes with a very low ratio of body fat to total body weight (see below).

BEING A THIN HARDCORE ATHLETE

The combination of very low body fat and the stress of competition may suppress menstruation completely. In addition, female athletes who participate in sports that value slenderness are more likely to develop serious eating disorders. These women may also suffer from osteoporosis, which is the loss of bone mineral density. Those most affected are runners, swimmers, gymnasts, and ballet dancers.

WEIGHT GAIN OR LOSS

Being either too skinny or too heavy can affect your menstrual cycles. Extremely thin teenagers and women, particularly those with the eating disorder anorexia, often stop having periods for months or longer. Those who lose 10 to 15% of their total body weight (or about one-third of their body fat) may also cease having periods. Finally, and as mentioned previously, female athletes often stop menstruating due to their low body fat.

On the other end of the spectrum are those who tend to be overweight. Excess fatty tissue can cause too much estrogen, disrupting the hormonal feedback system that tells the egg follicles to mature.

MEDICAL CONDITIONS

In addition to the various temporary factors listed above, a variety of medical disorders may cause women to stop ovulating indefinitely, including such things as thyroid conditions and pituitary tumors.

POLYCYSTIC OVARIAN SYNDROME (PCOS)

Although not that common in teenagers, all girls should be aware of this hormone condition, because it affects about 5–10% of all women. Some of the more obvious symptoms to look for are: obesity, excess facial and body hair, acne, and irregular cycles that continue at least two years beyond a girl's first period.

PREGNANCY AND BREASTFEEDING

Once a woman becomes pregnant, she cannot ovulate again until after the baby is born. This is so that her body can focus on nourishing the fetus within. And if she is breastfeeding, she can go for months without ovulating.

PERIMENOPAUSE

As women approach 50 years of age, they may stop ovulating as regularly as before. When they eventually stop releasing eggs altogether, they have reached menopause. Be aware, though, that a woman's fertility may significantly decrease already in her 30s.

Being Cycle Cautious

As you can see, there are many reasons why your cycles may be irregular at certain times in your life. But it's always a good idea to get checked by a gynecologist the first time you go a few a months without a period, just to confirm that there isn't a more serious underlying problem.

❋ THE "BIODRAMA" OF CONCEPTION AND PREGNANCY

My hunch is that at this point in your life you don't have plans to get pregnant anytime soon! I'm assuming that you probably aren't feeling particularly ready for the responsibilities of motherhood yet. And some of you may never want to be responsible for a baby's physical, emotional, and financial needs. However, you should know the basic biology of fertilization, especially since you now understand that everything about your cycle is ultimately geared toward a successful pregnancy.

Fertilization is the process of a man's single sperm burrowing into a woman's egg in order to form an embryo. Conception takes place in the outer third of the fallopian tube within a few hours of ovulation (it does not take place in the uterus, as many people mistakenly believe). The lucky sperm that eventually fertilizes the egg will have been victorious in its own biological race, in that perhaps 200 million or more of its tiny little siblings had set out with the same reproductive goal. It may travel up to several hours to reach its cherished date, and in fact, since sperm can live up to five days or longer in a woman's reproductive tract, the little guys may just "hang out," waiting to pounce once ovulation occurs. Yep, reproductive biology can be truly romantic.

In any case, once an egg is fertilized, it travels to the uterus with the help of vibrating cilia, which are hairlike projections that line the fallopian tubes. After a week or so, it will reach its ultimate destination of the uterine lining, where it will hopefully find a snug and cuddly home for the remainder of the pregnancy.

Once the embryo is safely burrowed into the uterine lining, the body's response is simply awesome. Since it would be disastrous for the endometrium to begin to disintegrate and shed in the form of menstruation (as it does in a normal cycle), the pregnant body has to prevent that from happening. But how? The newly embedded egg starts releasing a pregnancy hormone called HCG (which obviously stands for human chorionic gonadotropin!), which sends a message back to the corpus luteum left behind on the ovarian wall. Remember, the corpus luteum is the egg's casing that pumps out progesterone, thickening the uterine lining in preparation for the fertilized egg's soft landing.

The HCG signals the corpus luteum to not fizzle out, but to remain active several months beyond its normal maximum life span of 16 days. This will allow it to continue releasing the necessary progesterone to maintain the endometrial lining, which continues to nourish the embryo. About three months into the pregnancy, this task is taken over by the fascinating placenta, a temporary organ that develops during pregnancy in order to supply the fetus with all the oxygen and nutrients it will need until it's finally born.

OVULATION AND FERTILIZATION

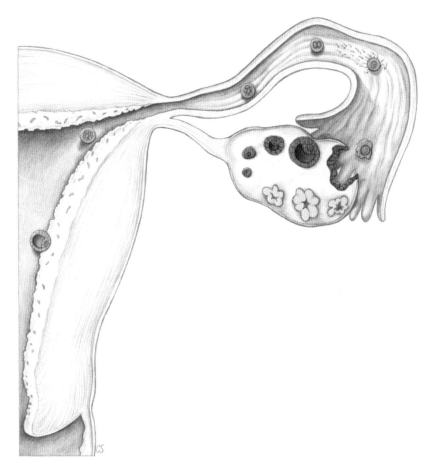

The life of an ovum

In the illustration above, a tiny egg within the ovary slowly develops its own follicle (red.) After completely maturing, it bursts out of the follicle and through the ovarian wall, in the most significant event of the menstrual cycle: ovulation. In most cases, the just-released egg (blue) will continue on its journey, moving forward through the waiting fallopian tube.

The follicular material left behind in the ovary will soon form the corpus luteum (yellow), which omits progesterone. If fertilization does not occur, it will die within 12–16 days, causing progesterone levels to plummet and menstruation to follow.

If intercourse occurs in the short fertile phase surrounding ovulation, the sperm will meet the newly released egg within the fallopian tube, where conception takes place. The fertilized egg would then continue the journey, implanting in the lining of the uterus about a week later.

Fertility Decreases as Women Get Older

You may be surprised to learn that a woman's fertility decreases as she ages. Even though a woman won't typically stop menstruating until she is about 50, her fertility starts to decline about 20 years before! In fact, female fertility peaks in the mid-20s, starts to fall in the 30s, and plummets in the 40s. There are several reasons why:

- Women are born with all the eggs they will ever have, so their eggs are as old as they are, and prone to chromosomal abnormalities as they age.

- The odds of the fertilized egg surviving implantation decreases the older it is.

- The quantity and quality of fertile cervical fluid tends to decline as women get older (more on cervical fluid in the next chapter).

- The older a woman is, the more likely she is to have any number of potentially fertility-compromising conditions such as endometriosis, PCOS, or fibroids (see Glossary).

- As women enter their late 30s, they tend to have more anovulatory cycles (cycles in which an egg is not released), and often those cycles in which ovulation does occur have shorter luteal phases (the phase from ovulation to menstruation).

The reason I address the issue of aging and fertility is not to scare you into having children sooner than you are ready! Rather, it is to educate you about all facets of your reproductive health, so that you can make informed decisions as you grow older.

✳ RETHINKING YOUR PERIOD, CYCLE, AND BODY

Whether or not you'll ever want to get pregnant, I hope these last few pages have convinced you that your menstrual cycle is an incredible example of the wonders of human biology, and despite what you learned when you were a kid, it's about so much more than just your period! The bottom line is that your cycles revolve around ovulation, not menstruation, and again, this is for a very simple reason: Every time you ovulate, your body is preparing for a potential pregnancy. As extraordinary as this is, I hope you would agree that this is reason enough to understand what's going on inside you!

Fortunately, that wondrous body of yours sends out a variety of remarkable signals that allow you to keep track of what's happening in your cycle, and more specifically, when you are about to ovulate. And as you will learn in the next couple of chapters, it is in observing these signals that you will truly become cycle savvy.

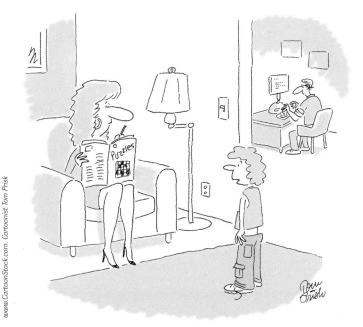

www.CartoonStock.com. Cartoonist Tom Prisk

"Thank goodness you were wrong mom, dad says a period is what comes at the end of a sentence."

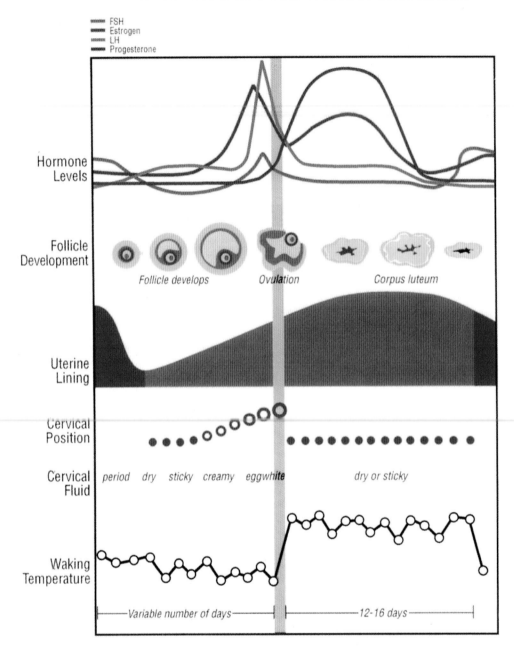

Note that the length of the phase before ovulation can vary widely, but the phase after ovulation is almost always 12 to 16 days. Within individual women, postovulation is remarkably consistent, usually not varying more than a couple of days or so.

Also note that the cyclical changes of the cervical position, cervical fluid, and waking temperatures seen on the bottom of this graphic are all discussed in the following chapter.

1. The main event of every cycle is
   a. *ovulation*
   b. *fertilization*
   c. *menstruation*
   d. *none of the above*

2. If a woman ovulates but does not get pregnant, when will she get her period?
   a. *The next day*
   b. *About two weeks later*
   c. *A month later*
   d. *She may not get her period.*

3. If a woman has cycles that vary between 24 and 36 days, does she need to see a doctor?
   a. *Yes*
   b. *No*

4. Ovulation occurs
   a. *on Day 28*
   b. *on Day 14*
   c. *during menstruation*
   d. *It can vary from cycle to cycle*

5. The factor that determines the length of your cycle is
   a. *when you get your period*
   b. *when you ovulate*
   c. *when you get PMS*
   d. *when your period stops*

6. If you got your period on January 1 and again on January 26, then your cycle length would be this many days:
    a.   25
    b.   26
    c.   27
    d.   28

7. What days is it normal to experience some spotting?
    a.   *After your red flow of menstrual bleeding ends*
    b.   *Around ovulation*
    c.   *Both of the above*
    d.   *Neither of the above*

8. Is it normal to have somewhat irregular cycles when you first start having your period?
    a.   *Yes*
    b.   *No*

9. If you have wildly irregular cycles that don't become regular after about two years of having periods, what might you want to get checked for?
    a.   *A vaginal infection*
    b.   *Diabetes*
    c.   *PCOS (polycystic ovarian syndrome)*
    d.   *A bladder infection*

10. Which of these variables can affect your cycle?
    a.   *Stress*
    b.   *Excess exercise*
    c.   *Gaining too much weight*
    d.   *All of above*

part two

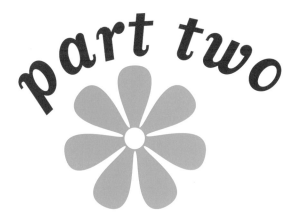

CYCLE
SIGNALS

a thing or two you can teach your mom

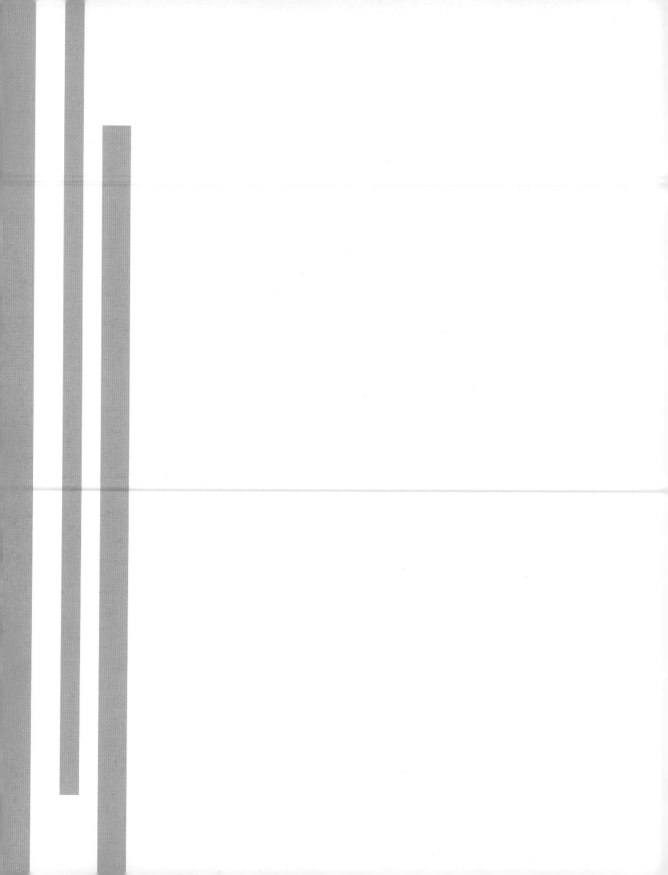

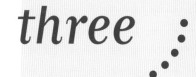
YOUR TWO FERTILITY SIGNS

at this point, you may be saying to yourself, "Wow, that last chapter was *way* more than I wanted to know about my body." And as you begin reading this one, you may be thinking, "I'm still a teenager and obviously not trying to get pregnant, so why is she going to teach me about my fertility signs?" Fair enough. But you'll soon see that these signs give you so much more useful information about your day-to-day life than just when you are fertile!

By learning how to chart your fertility signs, you can accurately determine not only when you are ovulating, but also other practical things about your body, like

* when your next period is *really* due!
* why your cycles are not always 28 days
* why your cycles may be irregular
* why you sometimes find secretions on your underwear
* why you "seem" (hmmm) to get vaginal infections every month

* why you "seem" (hmmm, again) to get periods every two weeks
* why your breasts sometimes feel sore
* why you sometimes feel like you've peed in your pants
* why you may crave fries or chocolate before your period

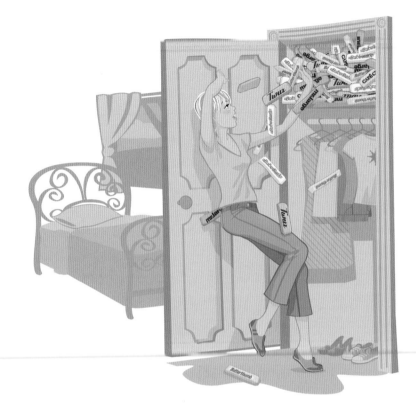

In brief, your body gives you all this information by providing you with two fertility signs that virtually all ovulating women experience: changes in waking temperature and changes in cervical fluid. In the next few pages, you're going to learn some fascinating things about the way these signs provide you with a secret window into what is really happening in your body between your periods. Then the next chapter will give you the tools to actually chart them for yourself. So let's get started with the two main fertility signs.

✳ WAKING TEMPERATURE

One of the most interesting things you can observe about your body is the pattern of your waking temperatures before and after you release an egg each cycle. You'll notice that upon waking, your temperature is much lower than you would expect. Before ovulation, your temperatures when you first wake up in the morning are relatively lower than normal. But after ovulation, your temperatures will usually rise and stay higher until your next period, about 12 to 16 days later. If you were to become pregnant, they would remain high throughout most of your pregnancy.

Waking temperatures within a cycle generally look like Anna's chart below:

TYPICAL WAKING TEMPERATURES

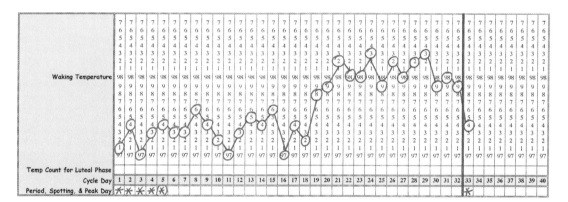

Anna's chart: Day 1 of Anna's chart is the first day of her period. This cycle length is 32 days, since she got her next period on Day 33. So she drew the closing vertical line just before the first day of her next period. Note that her temperatures show a pattern of two ranges throughout her cycle. In this particular cycle, on Days 1–18, her temperatures range between 97.0 and 97.6. On Days 19–32, her temps range between 97.8 and 98.3.

Your temperatures typically rise within a day or so after you ovulate (thus, ovulation most likely occurred on Anna's Day 17 or 18 above), and are the result of the heat-producing hormone progesterone. As you'll recall, progesterone is released by the corpus luteum, the remaining follicle on your ovarian wall that had surrounded the egg before it burst out of your ovary. So usually, the rise in temperature tells you that you have *already* ovulated.

✿ Average Waking Temperatures

Before Ovulation: 97.0–97.5°F

After Ovulation: 97.6–98.6°F

Certain factors can increase your waking temperature, such as:

* having a fever
* getting less than three consecutive hours of sleep before taking it
* taking it later than you usually do
* using an electric blanket, which you normally don't use
* drinking alcohol the night before

How To Prevent an "Uh-oh, I Just Got My Period" Moment

If you were to gather a group of women together, most could probably entertain you with countless tales of that surprise period that just came out of nowhere, or the one that seemed to be weeks "late" before it thankfully arrived.

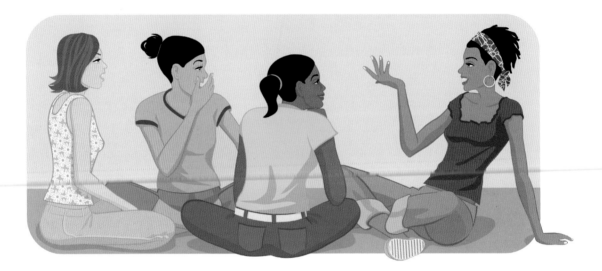

One thing you could be pretty sure of: They probably did not chart their cycles, because if they had, they would have known when to expect that first day of bleeding!

Well, this didn't happen to me (no, really!) but it was so embarrassing that I still think about it today. A bunch of us (guys, too) were sitting cross-legged just hanging out in my neighbor's den. She was sitting directly across from me wearing white pants, when a huge circle of blood soaked through. I'm sure everyone noticed, but none of us had the heart to say anything. She probably just died when she finally went to the bathroom. I think if that happened again today, I would try to quietly get her attention, because I would want someone to do the same for me.

—Mikela, 17

Charting your waking temperatures is the most effective way to know when your period is actually due. This is because your temps can help you identify if you've had an early or delayed ovulation, which in turn would cause your cycle to be shorter or longer than normal. Remember, once the temperature rises, it is typically a consistent 12 to 16 days until you get your period. And after you've charted for several months, you will be able to determine even more accurately what your own normal range is after ovulation. That's because for most women, the phase after ovulation doesn't vary by more than a couple of days.

SEEING THE FOREST THROUGH THE TREES

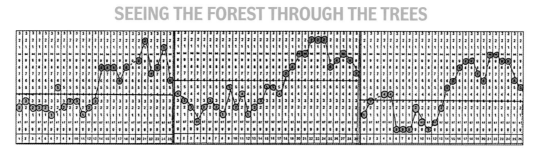

Note the obvious pattern of temperature shifts indicating ovulation in three of the author's charts, placed side by side. Even though there are a few temperatures that appear out of line or even missing, you can clearly see a pattern of lows before ovulation (blue) and highs after ovulation (red).

✳ CERVICAL FLUID

Have you ever taken off your underwear before your shower and been mortified to discover sticky, gooey stuff on them? If you're like most girls, you probably tried hiding them under the pile in the hamper, right?

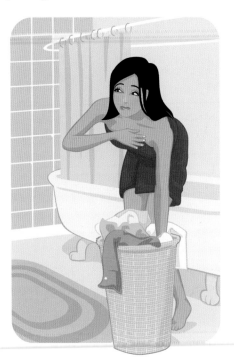

The good news is that what you've most likely been seeing is called cervical fluid, and it is a perfectly normal sign of a female body that is totally healthy and working as it should! In every cycle, your cervix (the opening of your uterus) produces a secretion that gets wetter and wetter as you approach ovulation. The specific purpose of this cervical fluid is to provide a substance in which sperm can swim to reach the egg around the time it is released.

Of course, at this point in your life, it may seem totally unnecessary and even bizarre for your body to go through this process if it doesn't need to, but remember, the entire menstrual cycle is the body's way of preparing for pregnancy. In fact, a pretty cool analogy of how your body prepares for a potential pregnancy every cycle is to think of how a seed germinates. When the ground is dry, the seed can't grow. But when the rain comes, it prepares the soil for the seed to sprout. Likewise, when you don't have any cervical fluid, or it is sticky, your eggs have not yet matured. But once you start producing wet cervical fluid, your eggs start developing in preparation for their release.

TYPES OF CERVICAL FLUID AS WOMEN APPROACH OVULATION

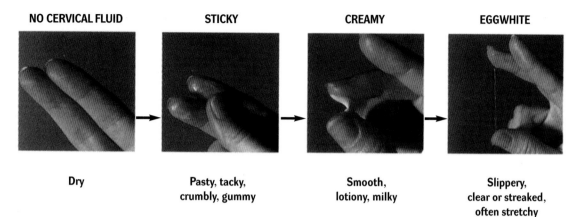

NO CERVICAL FLUID	STICKY	CREAMY	EGGWHITE
Dry	Pasty, tacky, crumbly, gummy	Smooth, lotiony, milky	Slippery, clear or streaked, often stretchy

Most women tend to be dry for a few days after menstruation, but as they approach ovulation, their cervical fluid becomes increasingly wetter. The above photographs show a typical pattern. A woman's Peak Day of fertility is the last day of a slippery, lubricative-quality cervical fluid or vaginal sensation. In the photos above, the Peak Day is the furthest right.

Some Tantalizing Tidbits About Cervical Fluid

- Men are fertile every day; therefore, they produce the substance for sperm to swim in, called seminal fluid, every day. Women, on the other hand, are only fertile during the few days around ovulation; therefore, they produce the wet, fertile cervical fluid for sperm to swim in only during those few days.

- Fertile cervical fluid functions exactly like seminal fluid. It assures that sperm can survive in an otherwise acidic vagina. In addition, it provides nourishment for the sperm and a substance in which they can swim toward the egg.

- This slippery-quality cervical fluid should not be confused with the clear lubricative substance that women produce only when they are sexually aroused (see page 60).

Once you start actually paying attention to these secretions, one of the first things you'll probably notice is the distinct pattern of cervical fluid you produce throughout your cycle. After your period, it typically starts to evolve in the following way:

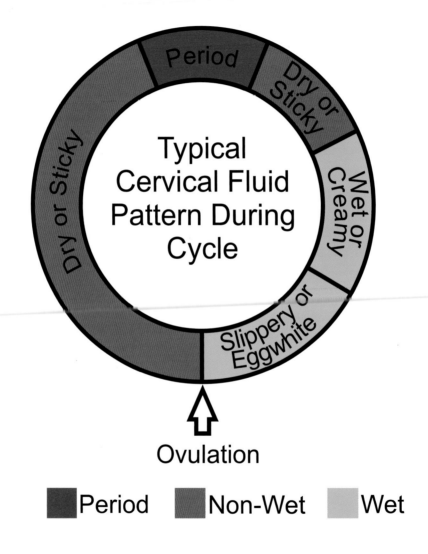

Can you think of what the significance is of the colors above?
Hint: check out the last paragraph of page 44.

In other words, right after your period, you may have a very dry vaginal sensation and observe *nothing* from your vaginal opening. Or you may notice a slight moisture similar to the way it would feel if you touched the inside of your cheek for a second. Your finger would have a dampness on it which would evaporate within a few seconds. This is the way the vaginal opening typically feels when there is no cervical fluid.

After perhaps a few days of dryness, you may begin to develop a type of cervical fluid that is best described as *sticky,* because it's like the glue or paste you used in elementary school. Occasionally, it may even seem like drying rubber cement, somewhat rubbery and slightly *springy,* but the important point is that it is *not wet.*

The next type of cervical fluid you may notice for several days is smooth, *creamy,* or lotionlike. It tends to feel rather cold at the vaginal opening, just as hand lotion feels cool to the touch. Sometimes this type of cervical fluid is so wet or watery that it is hard to physically handle (with a consistency similar to skim milk).

Finally, the most fertile-quality cervical fluid usually appears in the two to four days immediately before ovulation. It is the most noticeable type because it looks and feels like raw *eggwhite.* It's extremely slippery and may even stretch several inches. It's usually clear or partially streaked. It may even leave a fairly round pattern of fluid on your underwear, since it contains so much water. The most important point about it, though, is that it is very slippery.

CERVICAL FLUID ON UNDERWEAR

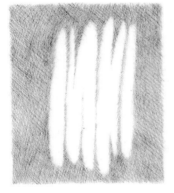

Nonwet-type cervical fluid tends to form more of a rectangle or line on your underwear.

Cervical fluid around ovulation often forms a fairly round circle, due to its high concentration of water.

What is so incredible about this slippery, eggwhite-quality cervical fluid is what it looks like under a microscope. Just look at it magnified in the picture on the following page, and tell me that isn't beautiful! Quick—what does it remind you of?

MAGNIFICATION OF CERVICAL FLUID

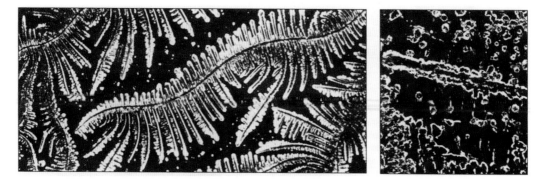

Fertile quality   Non-fertile quality

If you said a fern, you're right! Hopefully, after studying this gorgeous picture, you will develop a whole new perspective about that slippery stuff you sometimes feel when you wipe yourself after peeing!

After ovulation, your cervical fluid will usually dry up very quickly, and either disappear completely or maintain a sticky quality until your period. In other words, it may take up to a week for the fertile-quality cervical fluid to build up, but then it will usually dry up in less than a day. This sudden drying of the cervical fluid is one of the best ways to know that your egg has probably been released.

In general, most women will have no wet cervical fluid for the rest of their cycle. However, in the day or so before menstruation, you may occasionally notice a very wet, watery sensation, which may even resemble eggwhite again. This is absolutely normal, but can be a little confusing if you run to the bathroom expecting to find menstrual blood and discover this clear wetness instead! The moisture is actually caused by the water in the lining of your uterus beginning to shed, and thus you can be pretty sure that your bleeding will start within a day or so.

As with your waking temperatures, you should be aware that there are certain factors that can possibly mask cervical fluid. Among these are:

* vaginal infections
* antihistamines (which can dry it)
* sexual arousal fluid
* seminal fluid
* spermicides and lubricants

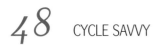

The Difference Between Healthy Cervical Fluid and Those Much-Dreaded Vaginal Infections

Almost every woman will get a vaginal infection at least once in her lifetime, and often many more times. Oh, goody. Since one of the classic signs of an infection is a vaginal discharge, how can you tell the difference between that and healthy cervical secretions? Actually, it's easy!

The beauty of charting your cervical fluid is that you will be able to distinguish what's normal for you from the nasty symptoms that result from a true infection, which typically include:

* abnormal discharge that may be green, foamy, or lumpy like cottage cheese
* an unpleasant odor or a yeasty smell
* vaginal itching, stinging, burning, swelling, or redness
* blisters, warts, or chancre sores

Understanding this distinction between healthy cervical fluid and vaginal infections is one of the most practical benefits you will gain from charting. In fact, it's very possible that your own mom or grandmothers endured unnecessary anxiety, made needless doctor appointments, and wasted countless dollars, all because they were never taught this basic biology. Thankfully, things will be different for you.

Now that you know the difference between healthy and unhealthy vaginal secretions, you can take control by immediately seeing a health practitioner at the first sign of an infection. After all, who wants to be miserable if they don't have to be!

My Cervix Does What?!

Who knew? Even your cervix, the lower part of the uterus that extends into your vagina, goes through some remarkable changes throughout your cycle. As with cervical fluid, the cervix itself prepares for a pregnancy every cycle by transforming into a natural gateway through which sperm can pass on their way to finding the egg. It does so by gradually becoming soft and open as ovulation approaches, in order to allow sperm passage through the uterus and into the fallopian tubes. Once ovulation has passed, it quickly returns to its usual condition of being firm and closed.

✳ SECONDARY FERTILITY SIGNS

Many women are lucky enough to notice other fertility signs that occur on a regular basis, all of which are very helpful in being able to further understand their cycles. They are referred to as secondary fertility signs, because they do not necessarily occur in all women or in every cycle for any individual woman. But these are still very useful in helping women to identify where they are in their cycle.

Secondary signs as ovulation approaches may include:

* ✳ ovulatory spotting
* ✳ pain or achiness near the ovaries
* ✳ increased sexual feelings
* ✳ fuller vaginal lips or a swollen vulva
* ✳ abdominal bloating
* ✳ water retention
* ✳ increased energy level
* ✳ heightened sense of vision, smell, and taste
* ✳ increased sensitivity in breasts and skin
* ✳ breast tenderness

The first sign listed above, ovulatory spotting, is a type of bleeding that may occur right around ovulation. It can range from just a tinge of red in the slippery fertile cervical fluid to bright red spotting for a day or two. Ovulatory spotting is more common in long cycles, and is caused by the sudden change in hormones at that time.

As for the various pains that women often notice around ovulation, there are several theories as to their cause, discussed on page 79. The important point is that you cannot say with certainty whether they are occurring right before, during, or right after you've ovulated. The pain may last anywhere from a few minutes to a few hours, and is usually felt on the side on which ovulation occurs. The typical pains are:

* ✳ dull achiness
* ✳ a sharp twinge
* ✳ crampiness

Now that you've learned about your fertility signs, the fun really begins. Once you read the next chapter, you'll probably never look at your body the same way again.

How cycle wise are you?

See How Well You Understood Chapter 3
Answers on page 177

CHECK THE VARIABLES THAT CAN:

AFFECT YOUR WAKING TEMPERATURE.

- ☐ Watching TV the night before
- ☐ Drinking alcohol the night before
- ☐ Inconsistent use of electric blanket
- ☐ Sleeping with your puppy
- ☐ Hot bath the night before
- ☐ Cold weather outside
- ☐ Less than three hours sleep
- ☐ Dreaming of figure skating
- ☐ Taking it later than usual

MASK YOUR CERVICAL FLUID.

- ☐ Vaginal infections
- ☐ Eating massive quantities of ice cream
- ☐ Sexual arousal fluid
- ☐ Cracking an egg in your underwear
- ☐ Sexual lubricant
- ☐ Spermicides
- ☐ Antihistamines
- ☐ Exercise
- ☐ Wearing shocking-pink-striped underwear

BE CONSIDERED SECONDARY FERTILITY SIGNS.

- ☐ Ovulatory spotting
- ☐ Brain meltdowns
- ☐ Depression
- ☐ Chocolate cravings
- ☐ Pain or achiness near the ovaries
- ☐ Fuller vaginal lips than usual
- ☐ An urge to dance

INDICATE A VAGINAL INFECTION.

- ☐ A squeaky-clean feeling
- ☐ Itching, stinging, burning, swelling, or redness
- ☐ Green, foamy, or lumpy discharge
- ☐ An intense desire to clean your closet
- ☐ The smell of fresh flowers in the spring time
- ☐ Clear, slippery, and stretchy secretion
- ☐ The smell of bread baking in your underwear

four

HOW TO OBSERVE AND CHART YOUR CYCLE

*n*ow that you've learned about your body's amazing fertility signs, you might be tempted to start observing them right away. The best way to do this is by charting, which is simply the daily observation and recording of your fertility signs each cycle. Why chart? Well, knowledge is power, girls, and with that knowledge comes pride instead of embarrassment, confidence instead of fear.

Look at it this way: If you had the lead role in a play and you didn't know half of your lines on opening night, you'd probably feel a bit uneasy on stage, perhaps even a bit freaked out and ashamed. In the monthly drama of your body's reproductive cycle, *you're* the lead. Charting is knowing your lines.

Take a peek at Brooke's chart on page 54. Now uncross your eyes—it's not as complicated as it looks! It's really a lot of fun. Brooke is feeling secure about herself because she knows, among other things, when she ovulated, when her period is due, how long her cycle is, what her vaginal secretions mean, how her life impacts her cycle, and how her cycle impacts her life. As the starring role in her body's drama, Brooke knows her lines!

You can, too. But I would encourage you to start out slowly. Maybe just *observe* your signs for a few months before you actually start charting what you've seen (although, if you're like a lot of girls, you may be really eager to just dive right in and chart!). Or maybe you'll want to focus on just one sign for a month or two, then the next sign. Of course, if you skip observing or charting now and then, it's no biggie. And don't get discouraged or bored if your charts don't necessarily look like those in the book. Sometimes it can take a few years for cycles to become regular if you are a teen, and until they do, you may not notice all the fun changes that occur with ovulating cycles. Eventually, though, observing your signs will probably become so routine that you'll just do it out of habit.

At this point you may be asking, So where do I begin? Hard as it may seem, the simplest way is to wait until the first day of your next period, which is the first day of red flow. Who knows? You may actually look forward to your period for the first time in your life!

Can You Chart While on the Pill?

If you are on the Pill, you won't be able to observe changes in your fertility signs, because the synthetic hormones in the Pill prevent you from ovulating. The only way you get to experience the cool changes your body goes through is if you have natural cycles.

❋ GENERAL CHARTING TIPS

* Make a bunch of copies of one of the two basic master charts on the last pages of this book, enlarging it by about 125%. The last page has some of the most common things you may want to record already listed on the bottom left (for example, feeling stressed, bloated, etc.). The other is blank for you to fill in yourself before making a bunch of copies. Or better yet, download the master charts from cyclesavvy.com!
* Punch three holes in the charts and insert them in a notebook devoted to your menstrual cycles. This notebook will become one of your most cherished possessions and a type of journal that you will undoubtedly refer to numerous times as you watch your cycles unfold over the years.
* Every period starts a new cycle, so take out a fresh sheet on Day 1 of your menstrual bleeding. Each page includes one complete cycle, from period to period.
* Fill in the top few lines above the temperatures as soon as you have Day 1 of your period, which is the first day of red blood flow.
* Each evening before going to bed, fill in your observations for that day.
* When you get your next period, draw a closing vertical line the day before. Repeat the first day of your period by transferring it to Day 1 of the new chart.
* Keep your most recent chart on top.

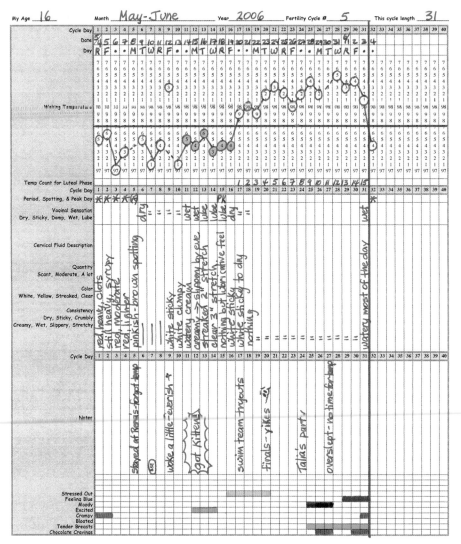

Brooke's chart: This cycle length is 31 days since Brooke got her next period on Day 32. So she drew a vertical line just after her last cycle day to show that it was a complete cycle from period to period. When she takes out a new blank chart for her next cycle, she will record Day 1 as the first day of red bleeding, and will repeat that one single day (June 4th, in this case) on that fresh chart.

Her wet cervical fluid on Days 11–15 warned her that ovulation was approaching, and her sustained temperature shift on Days 17–31 confirmed that she did, indeed ovulate. She counted 15 days of high temps after ovulation, and recorded them in the row just below her temps.

Notice how she uses lots of colors in the bottom rows of her chart to help her keep track of PMS and other events during her cycle, all listed on the left of the colored rows.

❋ WAKING TEMPERATURE

Taking Your Temperature

1. Take your temperature orally under your tongue every morning, first thing upon awakening, before getting up to use the bathroom (yikes), brushing your teeth, or even calling your best friend on the phone. But don't stress out. With a digital thermometer, we're talking about 60 seconds max, so it's really no big deal. Just set your alarm a minute earlier.

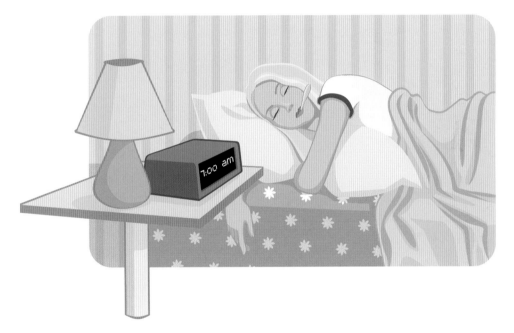

2. Take it about the same time every morning, within an hour or so. However, you don't need to be a slave to your thermometer. If you sleep in on the weekends, or for whatever reason you take it later or earlier, just be sure to note the time in the Notes section on your chart. This is important, because temperatures tend to rise a little the later you take them.

3. Try to take your temperature after you've had at least three hours of consecutive sleep. If you didn't, just note it on your chart.

4. Use an oral digital thermometer and wait until it beeps before removing it from under your tongue. If you prefer to use a glass one, it must specifically say basal body thermometer as opposed to a traditional fever thermometer.

Charting Your Temperature

1. Record your waking temperature by circling the ¹⁄₁₀th degree above either 97 or 98 degrees Fahrenheit. So, for example, if your temperature is 97.3, like on Day 1 in Carmen's Chart below, you would circle the 3 that is above the 97. (I know, I know, at first it sounds confusing, but trust me, it's a piece of cake.)

RECORDING WAKING TEMPERATURES

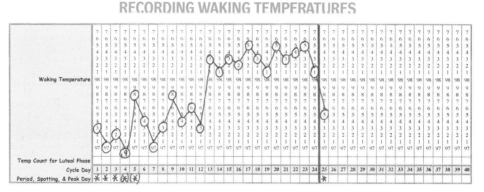

Carmen's chart: This cycle length is 24 days, since Carmen got her next period on Day 25. Her lower temperatures occurred between Days 1 and 12, and ranged between 96.9 and 97.8. Her temperatures then rose on Day 13, and remained high between Days 13 and 24, ranging between 98.1 and 98.5.

2. Record your temps with a pen, and everything else on your chart with a sharp or mechanical pencil, since you may want to occasionally erase the other notes. But if you think a temperature is outside the normal range (due to a fever or lack of sleep, for example), record it in *pencil* and wait until the next day before drawing the connecting lines. Omit the occasional outlying temp by drawing a dotted line between the normal temperatures on either side of them (see Daisy's Chart below).

RECORDING HIGHER-THAN-NORMAL TEMPERATURES

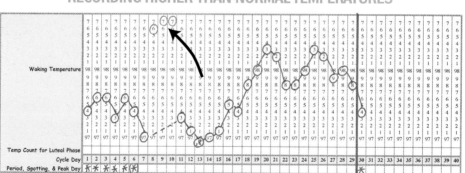

Daisy's chart: This cycle length is 29 days since Daisy got her next period on Day 30. Note how Daisy had a fever on Days 8–10, so her temperatures were clearly out of line. She circled the temps with pencil on those three days, then drew a dotted line on either side of them to indicate that they weren't part of her normal temperature pattern.

3. You should record unusual events such as stress, illness, moving, or travel in the Notes section at the bottom of the chart, and take them into consideration when interpreting your temperature pattern. After charting for a while, you'll see how life has a funny way of potentially impacting your temperatures. It's actually kind of interesting to predict when your temps may be affected by something. And be sure to include in this section whether you took your temperature earlier or later than usual (see Emma's Chart below).

RECORDING UNUSUAL EVENTS IN THE "NOTES" ROW

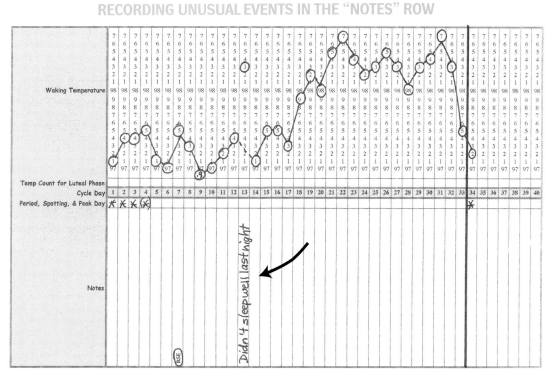

Emma's chart: This cycle length is 33 days since Emma got her next period on Day 34. Her lower temps ranged from 96.9 to 97.5. On Day 13, her temperature was abnormally high because she didn't sleep well the night before. She still circled her temperature, but drew dotted lines on either side of it. Then she had her true temperature shift on Day 18, after which her temps ranged from 97.9 to 98.7. (Curious about what that BSE is on cycle Day 7? Peek ahead if you'd like—the answer is on pages 88 and 89).

When Those Temps Just Don't Make Sense

You may notice that occasionally your temperatures are not that easy to interpret. In those cycles when you can't tell which day is the first day of a true temperature shift, you will love this great way to clarify things: draw a coverline, designed to separate the low temps before ovulation from the high temps after, as explained on pages 134 and 135.

A Word About Thermometers

- Make sure that your digital thermometer reflects temperatures only up to $^{1}/_{10}$th of a degree. For example, it should read 97.5 °F, not 97.54 °F.
- Digital thermometers beep when they have registered your temperature, usually within a minute.
- Glass *fever* thermometers? Don't even think about it. For one thing, they are *so* yesterday. And they are not accurate enough, because they only reflect temperatures to 2/10ths of a degree—for example: 97.2, 97.4, or 97.6 °F. Besides, they take longer and don't beep. Need I say more?

❋ CERVICAL FLUID

When you think about it, isn't it strange that by observing secretions from your vagina, you can determine when an egg the size of a pinhead is going to be released from inside your ovary? Well, as crazy as that sounds, it's a good thing that this fertility sign is so subtle. After all, things could be worse—imagine a NOW OVULATING signal flashing on your forehead instead!

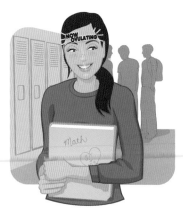

As you know now, virtually all ovulating women experience an observable pattern of changes in their cervical fluid throughout their cycles. Once they learn to recognize these differences, they usually realize how simple it really is to observe them. The bottom line is that when a woman is close to ovulation, her cervical fluid and vaginal sensation usually become wet and slippery.

A trick to help you identify the actual quality of the cervical fluid is to notice what it feels like to run some tissue or your finger across the bottom opening of your vaginal lips. Now don't be getting all squeamish on me at this point. Cervical fluid is natural, inevitable, and, for those who want to have kids one day, not even a fraction as frightening as what you'll one day discover in your baby's diaper! And remember, boys aren't all grossed out by touching their body parts, so why should you be?

In any case, when you use tissue to wipe near the opening of your vaginal lips, there are several questions you should ask yourself: Does it feel dry, preventing the tissue from easily moving? Is it smooth? Or does the tissue simply glide across? As you approach ovulation, your cervical fluid gets more and more slippery, and thus the tissue will just slide across easily.

Observing Your Cervical Fluid

1. Begin checking cervical fluid the first day after your period has ended.

2. Focus on vaginal *sensations* throughout the day (i.e., does the opening of your vagina feel dry, sticky, or wet? Does it feel like you are sitting in a puddle of eggwhite?). Vaginal sensations alone are extremely helpful in identifying where you are in your cycle, and doesn't even involve touching your vagina.

3. Notice your underwear throughout the day. Remember that very fertile-quality cervical fluid often forms a fairly symmetrical round circle, due to its high concentration of water. Non-wet quality cervical fluid tends to form more of a rectangular square or line on your underwear (see page 47).

4. Try to check cervical fluid every time you use the bathroom—at least three times a day, including morning and night.

5. *Before* urinating, separate your vaginal lips and feel your cervical fluid with your middle finger at the lower opening of your vagina or use a tissue to check, always wiping from front to back.

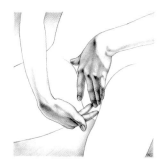

6. Glance away before looking at the cervical fluid so that you can really focus on its quality as you feel it with your fingers. Does it feel dry? Sticky? Creamy? Smooth? Slippery?

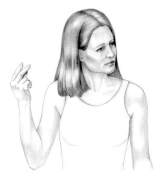

7. Look at it and note the color, consistency, and amount. Pay special attention to how slippery it feels.

8. Slowly open your fingers to see if it stretches, and if so, how much before it breaks.

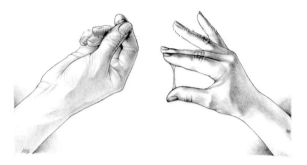

9. *After* urinating, focus on how easily the toilet paper slides across your vaginal lips when you wipe. Does it feel dry, smooth, or lubricated?

10. Pay special attention to cervical fluid after a bowel movement (I know, I know—*Eeeeeuuuu!*), since that is when wet-quality cervical fluid is most likely to flow from your vagina. Of course, to prevent infections, you must always wipe *from front to back* after using the toilet. Also, I hope it goes without saying that to further prevent a raging vaginal infection, you should use a different tissue to check your cervical fluid after going to the bathroom!

My aunt told me that she read about a girl who used to see that stretchy slippery stuff hanging from her vagina when she went to the bathroom, and was so confused by it that she would wad up toilet paper and aim it at it until it fell off, because she was afraid to touch it.

—Kisha, 17

Sexual Lubrication or Fertile Cervical Fluid— How Can You Tell the Difference?

Good question. Fertile cervical fluid tends to be thicker and remains on your finger until you wash it off. Arousal fluid tends to be thinner and typically dries quicker. And you'll only notice fertile cervical fluid for the few days leading up to ovulation. Still, one little piece of advice: You probably don't want to confuse things by checking your cervical fluid while daydreaming about that cute boy in your Spanish class!

1. Day 1 of the cycle is the first day of red menstrual bleeding. If you have brown or light spotting in the day or two before the flow, it is considered part of the previous cycle.

2. In the evening, record what type of bleeding and cervical fluid you noticed during the day. The adjectives listed in the box below are examples that can help you easily describe the types of cervical fluid you may notice.

Examples of Types of Cervical Fluid

Period	Red blood flow, syrup, clots.
Spotting	Carmel, brown, pink, or discolored (may occur around ovulation as well).
Nothing	Dry. No cervical fluid present.
	May feel dampness on finger that quickly disappears after you check.
Sticky	Opaque, white, or yellow, occasionally clear.
	Can be fairly thick. Critical quality is its stickiness or lack of true wetness. May be crumbly like paste, or gummy and springy like rubber cement.
Creamy	Milky or cloudy, white or yellow.
	Creamy or lotiony, smooth. Wet, watery, or thin.
	When separating fingers, may form small peaks of smooth lotion.
Slippery	Usually clear but can have opaque streaks in it.
	Very slippery and wet. Often causes extremely lubricated feeling at vaginal opening, but does *not* stretch like raw eggwhite below.
Eggwhite	Usually clear but can have opaque streaks in it.
	Very slippery and wet, like raw eggwhite. Often causes extremely lubricated feeling at vaginal opening. May stretch from one to several inches.

3. Record the most *fertile-* or *wet*-quality cervical fluid of the day, even if you are dry all day except for one single observation, as in Faith's chart below. (Any spotting should also be recorded.)

RECORDING CERVICAL FLUID

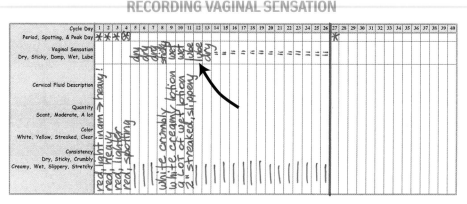

Faith's chart: This cycle length is 30 days since Faith got her next period on Day 31. Her period lasted the first six days, with spotting on Day 6. Then she didn't observe any cervical fluid until Day 10, when it started out sticky and got more and more wet as she got closer to ovulation. By Days 16 and 17, she had several inches of really slippery eggwhite-quality cervical fluid. But it dried up to merely sticky on Day 18.

4. Record the wettest vaginal *sensation* you notice throughout the day, since it is the most important indicator of where you are in your cycle. Don't be surprised if you have another day of a slippery or lubricative vaginal sensation even after the slippery cervical fluid itself has already disappeared, as in Gabrielle's chart below.

RECORDING VAGINAL SENSATION

Gabrielle's chart: This cycle length is 26 days since Gabrielle got her next period on Day 27. Her period lasted 4 days, with spotting on that last day. She didn't notice any cervical fluid for a few days after her period, but on Day 8, she started noticing cervical fluid that continued to get wetter through Day 12, after which it started to dry up. Notice that on Day 8, her *sensation* at her vaginal lips felt sticky, then wet for a few days. On Day 12, she recorded that her vaginal sensation was "lube" for "lubricative," even though her cervical fluid had stopped the day before.

✳ IDENTIFYING YOUR PEAK DAY

Once you have learned to chart your cervical fluid, you will want to use this information to dazzle your parents. Well, maybe not, but you will want to use your cervical fluid observations to determine as accurately as possible when you ovulated, and thus you will want to note the last day that you produced slippery cervical fluid *or* had a lubricative vaginal sensation for any given cycle.

This day is called the "Peak Day," because it is your peak day of fertility. It most likely occurs either a day before you ovulate or on the day of ovulation itself. The only way to know for certain would be to have an ultrasound done the moment the egg is released, and, well, I think you'd probably agree that it would be fairly impractical to keep an ultrasound machine conveniently located next to your bed.

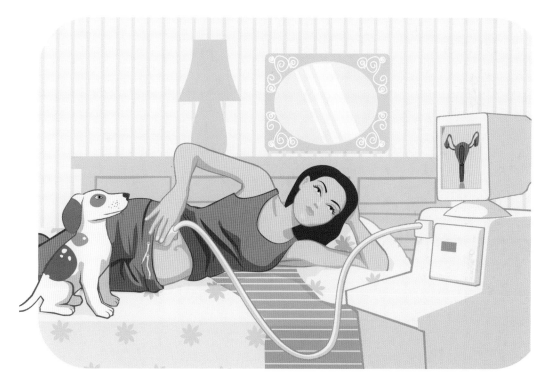

If you have really been paying attention, you should be thinking to yourself, "Wait a second! How can I know if I am experiencing my *last* day of wetness while it is happening?" Good point. You will only be able to determine the Peak Day after it occurs, on the following day. This is because you can only recognize the Peak Day *after* your cervical fluid and vaginal sensation have already begun to dry up. Then you can mark "PK" above it, as in Heather's chart on the next page.

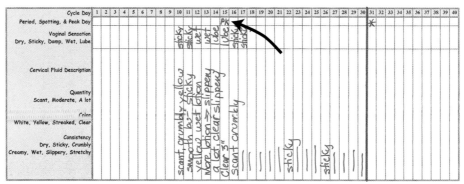

Heather's chart: This cycle length is 30 days since Heather got her next period on Day 31. Notice that she saw cervical fluid on Days 10 through 16. But the last day that she noticed wet quality cervical fluid or a lubricative vaginal sensation, was on Day 15, so that was her Peak Day. She marked it with "PK" just above that last day of wetness.

This idea of the Peak Day should become second nature fairly quickly. And practically speaking, it really doesn't matter if you can only identify your Peak Day on the day after, because it still tells you what you most want to know, which is the most likely day you ovulated. Again, that day is almost always the day of or the day after, your Peak Day, which is the last day you produced slippery cervical fluid *or* had a lubricative vaginal sensation. You are still fertile for up to a week before your Peak Day (and for some time after), but that one day is when you are the *most* fertile in any given cycle.

Your fertility, of course, may not be all that important to you at this stage in your life. Still, you'll be happy to learn that there are lots of other practical benefits to knowing when you ovulate, so stay tuned for the next chapter and you'll soon see why the information you're learning now will continually pay off, by taking the mystery out of your ever-changing body.

Appendix A: Keeping It Short and Simple

When you first learn about Fertility Awareness, it may feel more like work than fun. But soon enough, you may feel almost lost without the practical knowledge it provides you on a daily basis. Appendix A is a quick summary of everything you've learned about observing and charting your fertility signs, so you should refer to it often until charting becomes intuitive. See page 133.

✳ THE FUN OF CREATING A JOURNAL OF YOUR LIFE

Observing the changes in your cycles isn't just about waking temperatures or cervical fluid, or for that matter, even fertility or ovulation. In a very real sense, the charts that you create over the next few decades of your life will form the most intimate and practical diary that you could ever produce, because ultimately, they will serve as an enlightening window into the workings of your own body.

The practical everyday benefits will soon become evident, from knowing when to expect your period to being able to distinguish those gynecological phenomena that are both normal and cyclical from those that merit a trip to the doctor. And of course, if you do have to visit a physician, your charts will not only help her in treating you, but they will make you an active and informed participant in your own health care. Your charts, pure and simple, are self-knowledge, and as the saying goes, knowledge is power.

When you get older, you'll be able to see just how powerful these charts really are, since you'll be able to use them to effectively avoid pregnancy, or in reverse, to maximize your odds of getting pregnant. That's for later, though. In the meantime, you can begin this continuous and remarkably revealing journal, in which every chart will form a small chapter in your life-long journey as a healthy, empowered, and wonderfully self-aware woman.

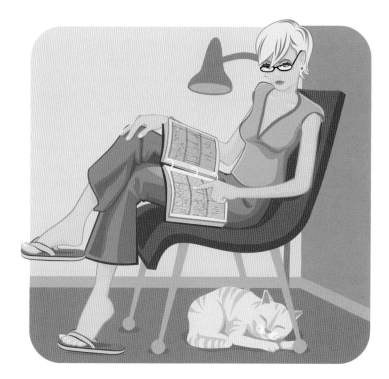

Are you cyclically empowered?

See How Well You Understood Chapter 4
Answer the questions on pages 67–69. Then record them across the rows
of this puzzle to discover the hidden phrase in the bold outline.
Answers on page 178.

1. The one day that is more fertile than any other day in the cycle:
   wet
   peak
   punk

2. The time of day when you should record the various fertility signs you noticed throughout the day:
   evening
   sunrise
   dusk

3. The best item in which to store your accumulating fertility charts:
   purse
   trash
   notebook

4. The feeling of your vulva around ovulation:
   cheerful
   wet
   sticky

5. The most important characteristic of your cervical fluid:
   quantity
   quality
   integrity

6. You should always be aware of this at your vaginal opening to help you determine your fertility:
   sensation
   condition
   restriction

7. The first day of the cycle is the first day of red _____.
   eyes
   cervical fluid
   bleeding

8. The moment that an egg is released from your ovary every cycle is when you are actually _____.
ovulating
menstruating
daydreaming

9. The purpose of drawing this line on your chart is to help you separate the low temperatures before ovulation from the high temperatures after ovulation, especially on charts where it may not be so obvious:
coverline
bottom line
online

10. The most fertile feeling you can experience at your vulva:
wet
lubricated
thrilled

11. The type of cervical fluid that is usually the *very first* indication that your estrogen is rising and you will be approaching ovulation:
sticky
creamy
funky

12. Each page of your fertility charts represents one _____ cycle, from period to period.
pathetic
partial
complete

13. You can predict when you will get this based on the consistent number of high temps that typically occur after ovulation:
blissful
infection
period

14. You should always take your temperature first thing upon _____.
   awakening
   sleeping
   eating

15. The most fertile-quality cervical fluid is _____.
   tacky
   creamy
   eggwhite

16. What that fertile-quality cervical fluid above often feels like between your fingers:
   sticky
   slippery
   butter

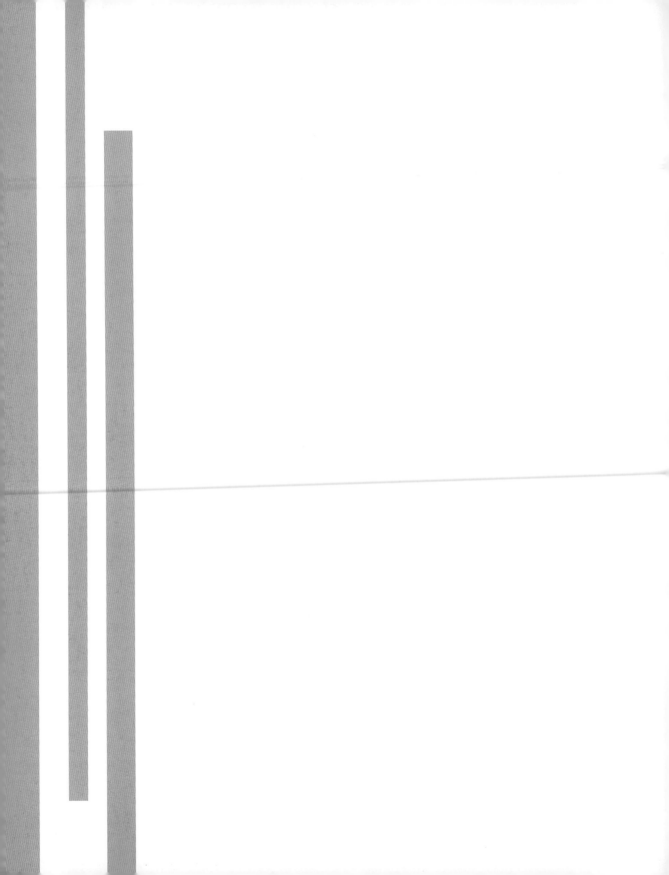

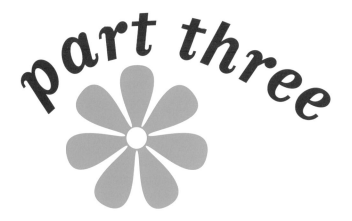

part three

CYCLE
SOLUTIONS

cool benefits of charting your cycle

OK, SO I'VE CHARTED.
NOW WHAT?

Once you've learned how to chart your cycles, the real fun begins. Maybe not the same kind of fun as in "Awesome, we're spending my 16th birthday in Hawaii" or "Wow, it's snowing and we've got the whole day off to party." Let's just say it's a more subtle and practical type of fun that will extend throughout your reproductive life. In fact, the most exciting benefits of charting are directly related to pregnancy (both avoiding and achieving it), but this will only be practical for you later in life, when you have a loving and long-term partner. Until then, though, there are still numerous benefits to charting your cycles, almost all of which involve finally understanding what your body is doing, why it is doing it, and whether it is normal. Consider the various female concerns that can now be demystified, all discussed in the following pages.

❊ PREDICTING YOUR NEXT PERIOD

Once you have identified when ovulation has occurred by your temperature shift and Peak Day, you can accurately predict when you will get your period. Charting your cycle removes the guesswork and allows you to plan ahead. Imagine the freedom of knowing whether or not your period will come over spring break—freeing you to show off that new little white bikini you just bought or, regrettably, to remind you to wear those crummy red shorts you've had forever.

> *Since I'm not sure when my period will come exactly, if I'm going to be in the water I always put in a tampon to be safe. But then it hurts when you take it out.*
>
> —Michelle, 14

Ouch! No wonder it hurts when Michelle takes out her tampon. Removing a tampon from a dry vagina is not only painful, but it can leave some tiny pieces of the absorbent material behind, causing a potential infection. Wouldn't it be nicer to just know when you are going to get your period? With charting, you can.

To determine when you'll start menstruating, just start counting from the first day of your temperature shift. Remember that the time from your first high temperature until your next menstruation is usually quite regular from cycle to cycle, not varying by more than a day or two. So, for example, if you usually have about 14 days from the first day of your temperature shift until your period, you may sometimes have 13 days or sometimes 15 days, but typically it remains really consistent. And if you are one of the lucky ones, you will also have even more advance warning by an obvious drop in temperature on the morning you start to menstruate. Of course, don't forget that as soon as you get your period, you should take out a clean chart, since the first day of bleeding becomes Day 1 of your new cycle.

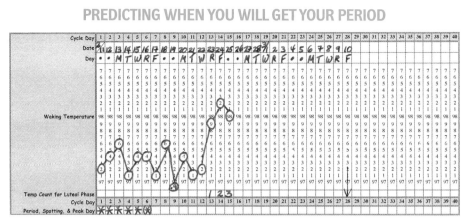

Isabella's chart: Isabella has noticed that she tends to have about 15 days from the first day of her temperature shift until she gets her next period. So once her temperature shifted on Day 13 and remained high for a few days, she counted ahead 15 days, drew a little arrow in pencil on the next day, and predicted that she would get her period around Day 28, or Marth 10th. How convenient is that?

✳ UNDERSTANDING THE DIFFERENCE BETWEEN HEALTHY CERVICAL FLUID AND ANNOYING VAGINAL INFECTIONS

Vaginal infections, especially yeast infections, are quite common, even in girls and women who aren't sexually active. If you haven't experienced one yet, you're in for a real treat—they're about as much fun as rolling in a patch of poison ivy.

The symptoms of a vaginal infection include any one of these signs:

* abnormal vaginal discharge that may be green, foamy, or lumpy like cottage cheese
* vaginal itching, stinging, burning, swelling, or redness
* unpleasant odor or yeasty smell
* painful urination

If you think that you have an infection, you should seek treatment as soon as possible. But it's unlikely anyone would need to persuade you. These types of infections are usually so uncomfortable that even immediate relief won't be soon enough. And if you're sexually active, avoid sex until it's gone!

OK, so that was the bad news. The good news is that charting your cervical fluid every day allows you to know your body so well that you can tell the difference between healthy cervical secretions and the symptoms of a true vaginal infection. Even better news is that there are many things you can do to avoid an obnoxious infection.

How to Avoid a Vaginal Infection

- Don't use harsh soap or feminine hygiene spray.
- Don't ever douche unless prescribed by a clinician.
- Bathe or shower every day, or at least after heavy exercise or anytime you get supersweaty.
- Wipe from front to back after using the toilet.
- Don't wear damp or tight clothes, because they can prevent healthy air circulation.
- Change your pads and tampons regularly.
- Always, always, always wear underwear with a cotton crotch, because cotton is a breathable fabric that limits bacterial growth.

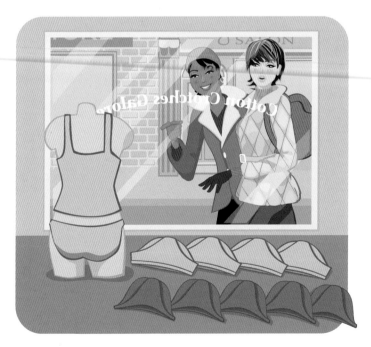

Normal Bleeding

It's important to know that not all vaginal bleeding is a period. Of course, if it starts as bright red flow and lasts about five days, most likely it is. But there are other types of normal bleeding that you should be aware of:

OVULATORY SPOTTING

As mentioned earlier, some women have a day or two of light bleeding right around ovulation due to hormonal fluctuations at that time. The spotting may be red, pink, or even brown, the color it becomes when it barely trickles out. Not only is this spotting normal, but it's another fertility sign that can help identify where you are in your cycle, as you can see on Day 20 of Jessica's chart below.

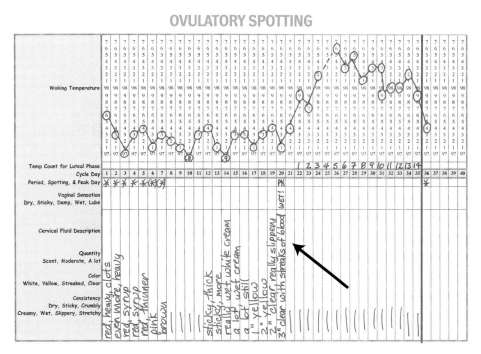

OVULATORY SPOTTING

Jessica's chart: This cycle length is 35 days since Jessica got her next period on Day 36. Her Peak Day was Day 20, the last day that she had a wet vaginal sensation and wet cervical fluid. Notice that on that day, she also experienced a little bit of pink blood mixed in with 3 inches of slippery cervical fluid, called ovulatory spotting.

ANOVULATORY BLEEDING AND SPOTTING

Occasionally women don't release an egg during their cycle, for any number of reasons, such as stress or illness. Again this is called an anovulatory cycle and may be longer than their usual cycle. When this happens, they may experience many days of spotting or even a heavier-than-usual period. The only way to determine if you have indeed released an egg that cycle is through charting your temperature. Remember, ovulatory cycles reflect a classic temperature pattern of lows before ovulation, followed by a consistent number of highs after. Kelly's chart below clearly shows anovulation by the lack of a temperature shift *that remains high* for at least 12 to 16 days before bleeding.

ANOVULATORY CYCLE WITH SPOTTING

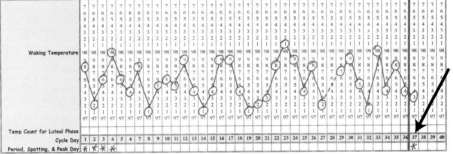

Kelly's chart: Notice that this particular chart is very different from others you have seen up until now because Kelly didn't have a temperature shift. This tells her that she probably did not ovulate this cycle. So even though this particular cycle length is considered 36 days because she started bleeding on Day 37, that bleeding (which can be just spotting) is technically anovulatory since she didn't ovulate this cycle.

SPOTTING AFTER OFFICE PROCEDURES

Women often spot after vaginal procedures such as Pap tests and pelvic exams, to name but a few. This is completely normal, and in the case of the Pap test is usually caused by slight irritation from the tiny brush used (see page 85).

SPOTTING WITH BIRTH CONTROL PILLS

Women who are on the Pill do not have true menstrual periods. It's only the withdrawing of the hormones during the fourth week of the Pill cycle which causes them to bleed. Also, women on the Pill often have spotting at different times during their cycle, none of which is a true period. This is called "breakthrough bleeding," and may be a sign that the particular Pill they are taking is not right for them, in which case they should consult their doctor. In any case, don't forget that women on the Pill won't notice changes in their fertility signs because the Pill is designed to prevent ovulation. If a woman *does* notice cyclical signs, it could be an indication that the pill is not working!

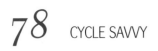

Blood clots during menstruation are common and are often more of a nuisance than a problem. One practical effect, though, is that they often make tampon use less efficient, because they block absorption and can cause leakage. Alas, this is not a pretty sight when you are wearing white pants! So if you find clots irritating and would prefer to try to minimize them, you may want to discuss this with your doctor.

Abnormal Bleeding

As you now see, different types of bleeding besides your period can be absolutely normal. However, if you have unexplained bleeding, you should seek medical attention just to rule out anything potentially serious.

Be particularly alert to such signs as cramping or abdominal pain, abnormal vaginal discharge, fevers and chills, or any kind of pain during urination or even sex. Such symptoms, when accompanied by abnormal bleeding, could be characteristic of a variety of conditions, from various sexually transmitted infections (STIs) to serious pelvic infections.

✳ UNDERSTANDING THE DIFFERENCE BETWEEN NORMAL CYCLE–RELATED PAIN AND ABNORMAL PAIN

Normal Cycle-Related Pain

Certain pain during a woman's cycle can be absolutely normal. For example, you may notice headaches in the postovulatory phase. If you find a *pattern* of headaches on your chart during only certain points in your cycle, you can be more confident that they are probably hormonally based, and this can help your clinician to work with you to treat them.

Another example of normal pain is ovulatory pain, which is thought to be caused by a number of factors, including:

* the follicles swelling within the ovaries
* the egg passing through the ovarian wall
* contraction of the fallopian tubes
* a small amount of blood being released into the pelvic cavity at ovulation

These are all considered normal causes of pelvic pain, and they can even be considered a secondary fertility sign. When you feel this type of pain, you can be pretty certain that ovulation is about to take place or has just occurred.

Abnormal Pain

On the other hand, if you notice pelvic pain that is intense or occurs at other times in the cycle, it could be an indication of any number of conditions that you should have checked to rule out any serious problems.

By accurately tracking your symptoms on your chart, you can help your doctor determine if you need further testing to diagnose the cause of the pain. For this reason, women should learn to recognize what is considered normal, cyclical pain as opposed to that which is more intense or occurs at unexpected times of the cycle.

Endometriosis

Endometriosis is an often painful condition that occurs when tissue that normally lines the uterine wall is found outside the uterus—usually in the abdomen, on the ovaries, fallopian tubes, or lining of the pelvic cavity. This misplaced tissue develops into growths, which respond to the menstrual cycle in the same way that the tissue of the uterine lining does. Each month the tissue builds up, breaks down, and sheds.

As you know, normally menstrual blood flows from the uterus and out of the body through the vagina, but the blood and tissue shed from endometrial growths has no way of leaving the body. This results in internal bleeding and inflammation—and can cause pain, scar tissue formation, adhesions, bowel problems, and infertility. Be aware, though, that in some women there may be no symptoms at all.

What Are the Symptoms of Endometriosis That You Can Chart?

- Pain before and during periods
- Premenstrual spotting
- Fatigue
- Painful urination during periods
- Painful bowel movements during periods
- Gastrointestinal upsets such as diarrhea, constipation, nausea
- Pain during sex

❋ BEING PREPARED FOR PREMENSTRUAL SYNDROME (PMS)

If you haven't already experienced PMS, not to worry. Your day will undoubtedly come. If you are like most women, you will probably have at least mild symptoms of it by the time you are in your mid-20s, and they may get worse as you get older or have kids. So what is PMS? If you've lived with your mother or sisters for any length of time, like oh, say, more than a month or so, you are probably fairly familiar with it already!

Whoever designed us thought it would be kinda funny to bless most of us with a bunch of annoying symptoms every cycle after we ovulate. What a comedian, eh? If you're lucky, though, you may get to breeze through your teens with few, if any, problems. But alas, your days of extended hormonal peace may be numbered.

Can You Think of Other PMS Expressions That Are More Accurate?

Pardon My Sobbing

Provide Me Sweets

Psychotic Mood Shift

Puffy Mid-Section

People Make me Sick

Pimples May Surface

Perpetual Munching Spree

Perennial Menstrual Syndrome

PMS Symptoms

The way symptoms are categorized varies among clinicians, though many tend to classify them into the four different groupings below. Still, be aware that most women don't necessarily fit neatly into any single category:

TYPE A—ANXIETY

Irritability
Mood swings

TYPE B—BLOATING

Weight gain
Breast tenderness

TYPE C—CRAVINGS

Cravings for sweets
Headaches and fatigue

TYPE D—DEPRESSION

Memory loss
Moodiness

Charting and Diagnosing PMS

To determine whether you have PMS, the most important thing is to see whether your symptoms are cyclical, meaning that when you get them, they are up to about a week or so before your period. The symptoms are caused by the hormonal changes that occur in an ovulatory cycle. So if you experience them both before and after you ovulate, they would *not* be considered PMS. And keep in mind that if you are not ovulating, you wouldn't experience classic PMS.

> *When I have PMS I just want to eat everything, even when I'm not really hungry.*
> —*Talette, 14*

When trying to determine if you have PMS, the first step is to chart your symptoms along with your fertility signs. By recording both, you can verify their cyclical nature and what factors may trigger them. Most women with PMS tend to notice the same symptoms from cycle to cycle. The best way to monitor them is to list them to the left of the narrow rows at the bottom of your master chart, as in Leah's chart on the next page. Most women who chart their cycles find that color-coding is a great way to immediately visualize when PMS symptoms occur in their cycle. Use colors that you associate with various conditions. For example:

Depressed	Blue
Chocolate cravings	Brown
Premenstrual cramps	Red
Irritable	Screaming orange (or some other obnoxious color)

Find colorful markers that are the perfect thickness for drawing lines on your chart. I personally use the ones called "Marvy Marker artist color 1300."

RECORDING PMS SIGNS

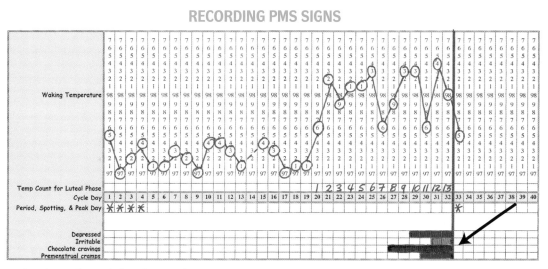

Leah's chart: This cycle length is 32 days since Leah got her next period on Day 33. Notice that about a week before she got her period, she started experiencing some fairly typical signs of PMS, such as feeling depressed or irritable, or having chocolate cravings (oh, yeah!). Recording premenstrual cramps may come in handy one day if she needs to discuss them with her doctor. As you can see, by making each symptom a different color, it makes the whole chart easier to interpret and a lot more fun.

Treating PMS

Once you have determined the cyclical nature of your PMS symptoms, you can then decide on the appropriate steps to take. Often the symptoms themselves create needless anxiety as women wonder if they are "going crazy" or suffering from a serious illness. Yet many women find that just being able to anticipate PMS symptoms will help them cope with them. When you realize that your depression, bloating, or irritability is only a sign that your period is a few days away, you should have less cause for concern. The knowledge and control that come with charting can be the first step in managing PMS. If you find, though, that your symptoms are more severe, you should discuss them with your health care provider. Of course, the fact that your charts detail which specific symptoms you have will help her to better treat you.

The simplest ways to deal with PMS are often found within your own body, and not in a medicine cabinet. For example, simply exercising three to five days a week, eating a healthy diet of fresh fruits and vegetables and lean meats, or practicing relaxation techniques can work wonders. And for many, specific vitamins and minerals may help, depending on what their particular symptoms are. There are loads of great books available on just PMS, so you can be sure it's a very common problem.

✳ BEING PREPARED FOR YOUR FIRST GYNECOLOGICAL EXAM

If you are like most teenage girls, you probably dread the idea of your first appointment with a gynecologist. That's only natural. I mean, let's get real—you'd probably rather be studying Latin than finding yourself with knees apart in front of a doctor you may never have even met before.

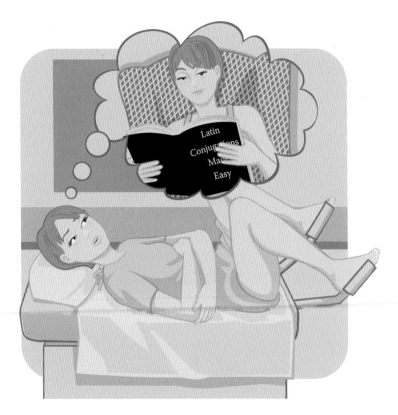

Part of your fear about the visit will undoubtedly be your sense of vulnerability. But imagine, instead, if you arrive feeling confident and knowledgeable because you've charted several cycles beforehand. More precisely, imagine how much easier it will be if you understand what your body is up to, as well as what the doctor will be doing during the exam.

With Fertility Awareness, you can become an active partner in your health care. And if you know ahead of time which procedures to expect, these exams won't feel so intimidating. For example, one of the purposes of an annual exam is to get a Pap test, in which cells from your cervix are collected to check for abnormalities.

Wouldn't ya know—the test we all love to hate so much is named after a man, Dr. George N. Papanicolaou, the doctor who developed it! So if you want to impress someone, try the receptionist, who may go cross-eyed the next time you try scheduling a Papanicolaou test. On second thought, maybe you'd better just stick to asking for a Pap test.

The ideal time to get it done is when you are approaching ovulation and your cervix is already open, since this makes it a lot more comfortable when the doctor inserts the tiny brush inside to swab some cervical cells. A tiny *what* goes *where*? Don't worry—for most women, the cervix has little or no pain receptors, so you'll barely feel a thing. With daily charting, of course, you'll know when you're near ovulation, and thus will have a greater ability to schedule the exam at the most comfortable time.

Who Performs Gynecological Exams?

Family practice physicians

Pediatricians

OB/GYNs

Medical assistants

Nurses

Nurse practitioners

Midwives

Naturopaths

Another purpose of the appointment is to get a breast exam to check for possibly abnormal lumps. It is better to avoid having this exam done in the week preceding your period, because your breasts are much more likely to be tender and already somewhat lumpy during that time. The bottom line is that knowing precisely where you are in your cycle will help you to schedule medical appointments at a time that is most comfortable for you.

What to Expect During Your Annual Gynecological Exam

Needless to say, this is not exactly every female's favorite medical appointment. At this point, you may be wondering if you really have to subject yourself to such seeming torment. Generally speaking, it's probably a good idea to get your first gynecological exam by about 16, or even younger if you are considering becoming sexually active or already are.

Yet rather than dreading it, why not think of it as an opportunity to take care of yourself and get all your personal questions answered in a completely safe and private setting? Of course, if possible, you may want to schedule your appointment with a female practitioner.

The purpose of this exam is to determine if your reproductive organs are healthy, and to detect any medical concerns such as infections or abnormal Pap tests. It usually consists of the following:

History taking: The clinician will ask you questions related to your family medical background, such as whether family members have had life-threatening health conditions. She'll also ask about your lifestyle, including such things as nutrition, exercise, and your recreational habits. In addition, she will ask you about your sexual history, including if you have had sex yet, what types of sex you engage in, how many partners you have had, and what you are using for birth control. She is not being nosy. She is being a good doctor. This is a great time to ask questions in a confidential environment, and to mention any health concerns you may have.

General exam: The clinician will check your blood pressure, thyroid, heart, lungs, and abdomen, and will probably examine your mouth and ears. She will do a breast exam to check for unusual lumps, and may even teach you how to do your own monthly breast exam, which women are encouraged to start doing in their early 20s. (See page 89.)

Pelvic exam: This is the part of the exam that will probably feel pretty weird, but just remember, your clinician has done this zillions of times, and will be completely professional about it. She will examine and feel the shape of your reproductive organs, including your vulva (your external area around your vagina), uterus, and ovaries.

During the internal exam, the clinician will ask you to scoot down as far as you can on the table, place your feet in stirrups, and let your knees fall to each side (I know, I know, this is hardly your idea of a good time. But maybe you can think of it as a unique new yoga position. Or not).

The practitioner will first look at your vagina for any sores or lesions, then separate your vaginal lips to gently insert a speculum, an instrument that will allow her to see and access your vaginal walls and cervix. Speculums are either plastic or metal and are similar in shape to a duck's beak.

The main purpose of expanding your vagina is to do a Pap test, in which a sample of cells is taken from your cervix so that it can be evaluated for any unusual changes. The cells are usually collected with either a tiny brush or a thin wooden stick. Truth be told, it's not the most pleasant feeling, but it lasts only a few seconds, and it shouldn't really hurt. Maybe feel awkward, yes. But not hurt.

And if you are sexually active, you should ask to be tested for STIs, even if you don't have symptoms. Some of the more important infections to be screened for are HIV, herpes, Human Papilloma Virus (HPV), chlamydia, and gonorrhea.

After the clinician removes the speculum, she may insert one or two fingers inside your vagina (while wearing gloves and using lubricant) to feel your uterus and ovaries. Don't be surprised if she also inserts a finger in your rectum while pressing down on your uterus. This helps her to stabilize your uterus and feel its position better. The internal exam itself is fairly quick and shouldn't be scary, but it might be a little uncomfortable. And for what it's worth, most clinicians will tell you that they don't like getting pelvic exams any more than you do!

One day, I thought I had an infection and had to go to the gynecologist on the heaviest day of my period. Even though my doctor tried to reassure me by insisting that she sees girls all the time during their period, I was still so embarrassed. Just as I scooted down, I dripped a huge drop of blood right on her white shoes! She just laughed, but I wanted to die.

—Caitlin, 18

✳ MAINTAINING YOUR HEALTHY BREASTS

You may have already noticed that your breasts can feel more tender in the latter part of your cycle, usually in the week before your next period. This is normal and is the result of hormonal changes that occur after ovulation. Even something as seemingly routine as taking a shower can be uncomfortable for you in the week before your period. Of course, showering with a shield covering your breasts may be a tad extreme!

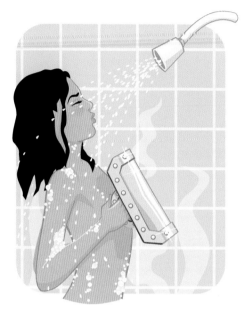

You may also have noticed that you tend to have somewhat lumpy breasts during this time. Again, this is usually nothing to be concerned about, and if this happens every cycle, you may well have what are referred to as fibrocystic breasts, or breasts that tend to develop small, fluid-filled cysts. You should have them checked by a health practitioner at least once when you feel the lumpiness, just to rule out potential problems.

One of the best routines you can get into for your long-term breast health is to do a monthly breast self-exam (BSE) on Day 7 of your cycle. The reason to check them on this day is that this is when your hormones are least active, so it is when you'd be able to most easily notice potentially abnormal lumps. Over time, you'll also begin to recognize how your own breasts normally feel. And while it is extremely rare for teenagers to discover a cancerous lump, getting into the habit of doing a monthly breast self-exam is a great lifelong practice.

A WOMAN PERFORMING A BREAST SELF-EXAM ON DAY 7 OF HER CYCLE

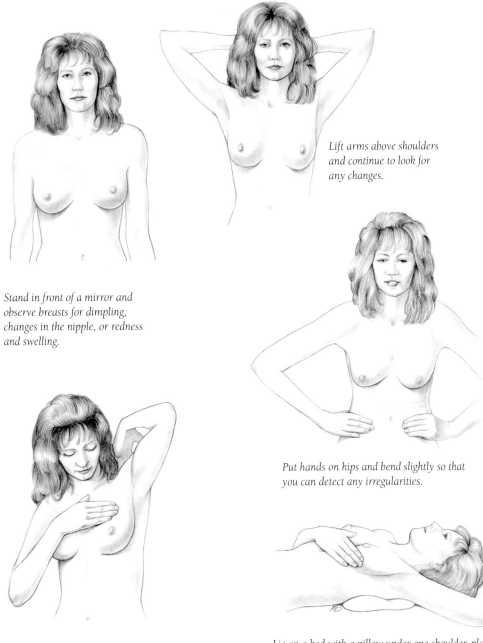

Lift arms above shoulders and continue to look for any changes.

Stand in front of a mirror and observe breasts for dimpling, changes in the nipple, or redness and swelling.

Put hands on hips and bend slightly so that you can detect any irregularities.

Check breasts while showering, using soap to help your hands glide over your breasts.

Lie on a bed with a pillow under one shoulder, placing your arm behind your head. Using the pads of your fingers, feel for lumps or thickening with the opposite hand.

Can you unravel the mysteries of your cycle?

See How Well You Understood Chapter 5

Answers on page 179.

Warning:
This quiz is a tad more challenging than the others,
but since just reading this book is making you so much wiser, you'll probably do fine!

CIRCLE THE WORD THAT DOES NOT BELONG.

1. increased energy • cervical fluid • ovulatory spotting • swollen vulva

2. around ovulation • while taking vitamins • after Pap tests • while on the Pill

3. headaches • breast tenderness • increased intellect • bloating

4. itching • swelling • clear and slippery secretion • unpleasant smell

5. Pap test • breast exam • possible blood test • manicure

6. menstruation • consistent length • high temps • PMS may occur

7. wear cotton crotches • don't douche • drink ice-cold lemonade • wipe from front to back

8. toe cramps • abnormal discharge • fever and chills • abdominal pain

9. follicles swelling • egg passing through ovary • a little blood released • fallopian tubes twisting

10. pregnancy achievement • natural birth control • gynecological health • menstrual elimination

six

NOW THAT YOU KNOW
From Cycle Savvy to Sex Smart

Congratulations! You've made it to page 91, hopefully still in one piece despite the, well, slippery subject matter. So why don't you step back now and see how everything you've learned so far fits together. What you discovered at the beginning of this book is that ultimately, your body prepares for a potential pregnancy, each and every cycle. In other words, the biology of menstruation is all about reproduction, and that, plain and simple, brings us to the subject of, yup . . . *sex*. Ah yes, the apparent obsession of every teenager and every teen's parents, but for ever-so-different reasons!

When I was 16, I brought home my first sort of serious boyfriend, just so that my mom could see I actually had good taste in boys. He was a year older, but he was shy and very sweet. In other words, very unthreatening, so I just didn't think there would be a problem. The thing is, he really liked me and I really liked him, and so naturally for mom, that was a big problem!

—Marti, 35

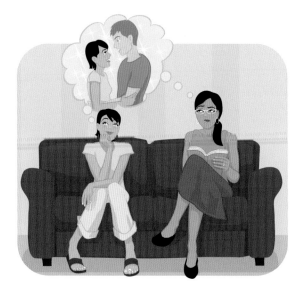

Before I even continue, I want to come clean with you about something. This has been a really difficult chapter to write, partly because the subject of sex is so often presented in ways that are either preachy, moralistic, or flat-out depressing. But that's just not my style, and it certainly won't change now. The reality is that sex can be awesome, but only at the right time, in the right context, and with the right person. And the one word that should always be at the center of any sexual decision is this:

Respect

Respect for your body, respect for yourself, respect for your partner, and perhaps most of all, respect for the potential consequences of having sex.

Around the age of 14, I discovered that my sexuality gave me some sort of power over guys, and I used it to make me feel better about myself for the 15 minutes or so that I was hooking up with a guy. I was his whole world. Yet I usually felt unsatisfied, both physically and emotionally.

The guy became a stud and I became a slut. I still felt lonely, I still felt empty, I still wanted to be loved. So I would end up doing it all over again. It took me almost five years to realize that, after those 15 minutes were up, I had actually given away my power by being with someone who didn't respect me. I really had to learn to respect MYSELF in order to retrieve it.

—Marie, 26

As you may already know from sex-ed classes, anything related to gynecological issues often includes a set of "watch-out-fors" and other cautionary messages. We're talking potential unplanned pregnancies, sexually transmitted infections (STIs), and that whole list of truly yucky downers. These messages are usually delivered by a much older adult, so the translation sometimes gets scrambled and all you hear is the doom-and-gloom-preaching "Don't-even-*think*-about-having-sex-until-you're-over-30" kind of message.

So let's make a deal. I'll spare you yet another dreary lecture, sure to leave your eyes rolling. You, on the other hand, need to know this material for your own knowledge, health, and sanity. I want to empower you with information, and then trust you to use that knowledge to take responsibility for your own body and life. I'm not going to sugarcoat anything, nor am I going to talk down to you. I assume that if you're reading this book, you are already smart and determined to make wise decisions that will be good for you today and in the future.

❋ HOW WILL YOU KNOW WHEN YOU ARE READY FOR SEX?

Wanting to have sex is a natural human desire. When you first start to think about your own sexuality, it's important to realize that all the conflicting emotions, cravings, and confusion that you may experience around sex are not only normal, but probably inevitable. After all, sex and its various related topics, from romance to fertility to homosexuality, are all complex matters that fill bookstore shelves everywhere. Having said that, one of the most important decisions you will ever make is when and with whom you choose to have sex.

Of course, before you even make that decision, you have to define for yourself what sex is. Some people think of it as only sexual intercourse. Others think of sex as anything that involves any kind of sexual touching, including being physically intimate with another person through oral sex or even just sleeping in the same bed with them. The point is that you can put yourself in a very vulnerable situation regardless of what type of sex you engage in. So here's a fundamental truth:

Girls have a lot more to lose from sex than boys do.

For starters, there's the obvious risk of an unplanned pregnancy, as well as the risk of contracting an STI that can lead to infertility. But those are just the physical consequences, and don't even include the emotional pain that can come with sexual misjudgment.

Ultimately, the goal of this chapter is to honestly explore things that you need to consider when deciding if you are ready for sex. But what makes this chapter completely different is that I got a lot of help from some female, well, co-authors . . . women who have already been there, done that. Read on and learn from their experiences, both positive and negative. For example:

> *When I was 17, I was dating a 19-year-old college student who was sexually experienced. I was not. He started asking me about having sex with him. He kept telling me how great it would be. I had friends who were sexually active so I thought that was what I should be doing. We set a date and time to have sex. I was really nervous about it. I really thought that I loved him, but I wasn't sure that I was ready.*
>
> *A friend of mine gave me the best advice—if I was having any doubts about wanting to be with him, then I shouldn't do it. I would regret it. Thankfully I listened to her. A few days before we were supposed to have sex, I told him that I had changed my mind. He got really angry with me and told me off. At that moment I knew that I had made the right decision. I broke up with him soon after and saved myself for someone when I was older!*
>
> —*Ava, 37*

Some of you will become sexually active before your friends do, while others will choose to avoid serious sexual activity until you're much older, or even married. Most of you are straight, but some of you will realize you're gay or bisexual. Many of you may already be extremely interested in sex, and others perhaps not at all. The point is that every person's sexuality develops differently and on its own timetable. The most important thing you can do for yourself is to develop an unwavering self-respect that will wisely guide you in deciding when and with whom to become sexually active.

❋ TAKING SEX SERIOUSLY: SOME THINGS TO CONSIDER

First and foremost, of course, is to accept that you are unique, both in terms of where you are now in your physical and sexual development, and the person you'll become as you grow older. So think about the following issues as you contemplate the question of when you will be ready for sex, or even whether you want to continue having it if you are already sexually active. In either case, you can take control of your sexual choices so that you maintain a healthier you—both physically and emotionally.

Your Personal Values and Goals

You can't escape it. Whether you were raised in a tree house, a traditional home, or somewhere in between, chances are you've been affected in many ways by the values of those raising you. Were you brought up in a religious household? In a liberal atmosphere? Were your parents open with you about their hopes and dreams for you? Even more importantly, what are your *own* hopes and dreams?

> *I understood that an unplanned pregnancy was the quickest means to derail my dreams of college and career. I never felt my virginity was a burden to unload.*
>
> —Martha, 39

As you can imagine, your goals in life can have a profound impact on your attitudes about so many things, including whether or not to have sex. For example, do you want to go to college and pursue a career or settle down soon after high school? Are you obsessed with art or travel or dance?

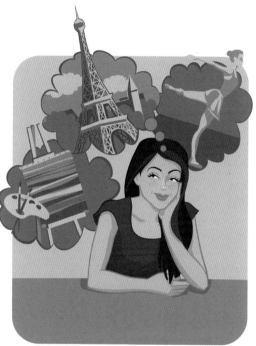

What are some interests that pull at your heartstrings? If you envision getting married shortly after graduating, you may feel very differently about when to start having sex than if you plan to pursue your passions, attend college, or start a career before settling down. One of the best things you can do to help you figure out if you are ready to have sex is to ask yourself *why* you want to do it. Out of curiosity? For the physical pleasure? Because everyone else is doing it? To express your love to your partner?

To help decide what is best for you, perhaps you should grab a journal and jot down the answers to these questions, as well as your personal values and goals. Later, you can add thoughts that come up as you read what the following women had to say on these very issues:

My boyfriend never pressured me. We took things sooo slowly. Discovering the alternatives to intercourse has its own rewards, believe me. By the time we were both ready to go all the way, it was such a sweet, gentle experience, with so much "warming up," there was absolutely none of the physical pain I know some women experience, and definitely none of the weird emotional feelings that so many of my friends had.

Pretty cool first-time experience! I know it has influenced all my relationships since. I have pretty high expectations for mutual respect, and anyone who doesn't meet them is quickly shown the door.

—Alice, 40

As a teenager you're often told to "wait until it is right" before you have sex. Such an open-ended statement. How do you know it is "right"? Until you're older? Until you're smarter? Until you're in love?

Well, in third grade I believed I was in love. By the time I got to sixth grade, I knew that my third-grade crush wasn't love, but my sixth-grade crush truly was! Obviously, by the time I was in high school, I knew those childish crushes weren't love, but this newfound feeling certainly was! You get the idea.

Each time, had I simply been waiting for the time to be "right," I would have made some irreversible decisions regarding sex. On my wedding night, when I was 27, I knew for sure that I'd made the right decision.

—Sonya, 33

My first experience with intercourse was when I was away at a six-week summer camp. I was 16, he was 19. He seemed very hurried, not at all romantic and loving. I think it was 10 minutes and he was out the door. I found out afterward that I was also his first, and his reason for having sex with me was that he was "getting older and wanted to know what all the fuss was about." It wasn't until a few years later that I had my first LOVING intercourse and finally knew what the fuss WAS about. Having sex for the wrong reasons is just that—wrong.

—Jennifer, 36

Your Willingness to Take Physical Risks

Of all the issues you need to consider, none are more widely discussed than the risk of unwanted pregnancies and STIs. While these are, in fact, huge social problems, the reality for you is much more personal and immediate. There are very real physical risks that come with being sexually active, so if you are, you need to know what those risks really are and how to keep them to an absolute minimum.

PROTECTING YOURSELF FROM UNPLANNED PREGNANCIES

(For specific information on birth control options, see Appendix C on page 149.)

Here's a humbling thought: You are more fertile in your teens and early 20s than you will ever be! That's a pretty profound concept when you think about it. Of course, I don't need to tell you what you have heard zillions of times before: The only 100% effective way to avoid an unplanned pregnancy is to not have sex, or more specifically, not to let those sperm get anywhere *near* your vagina!

My high school boyfriend and I had been dating for three years, the last one of which we were having unprotected sex. I loved him and thought we would be together forever. The thought of a child never entered my mind. We, of course, broke up.

I was probably five months along before I realized I was pregnant—probably due to the fact I was in denial and had very little clue about how my reproductive cycle worked. I was just 17 and knew a baby would only suffer the consequences of my mistakes. I was way too young to give a child all of the love, time, and attention he/she needed. Plus I wanted only the best for my kids and I needed to go to college for that. Why should my child suffer because of my stupidity?

So I opted for an open adoption. I felt like I could turn my mistake into someone else's blessing. While it caused me a lot of pain, I made two people's dream come true and that felt great.

—Jeni, 37

Upon turning 16, I decided that I was ready to have sex. Being sure that my steady boyfriend would be clueless and irresponsible, the first thing that occurred to me was that I should get outfitted with some sort of protection. So I took myself over to my family practitioner, a nice hippie doctor who was more than happy to prescribe me a diaphragm. I recall being simultaneously amused, horrified, and dubious as she explained how to operate the device. Nonetheless, I made it out the door, protection in hand, without bursting into tears or hysterical laughter. Looking back, I have no idea how I paid for this—did insurance cover it?

Next up was planning a special occasion. My boyfriend's parents were going out of town. Perfect. A dinner reservation at a nice restaurant. Perfect. A few practice tries at inserting the diaphragm. Not so perfect. It was slippery, springy, and completely unwieldy but I wrangled it into what I thought was the right place. Dinner ensued, romance happened, and my boyfriend was thrilled and then suddenly terrified and then back to thrilled. We fumbled around, had some awkward sex, and felt initiated. I felt satisfied and very proud that I had pulled the whole thing off safely so I could enjoy the experience without worrying about ruining my life with an unwanted pregnancy.

—Betty, 38

I became sexually active at the age of 15. When I was 16, I was involved with a boy at my high school. We were together about three months prior to having sex. We regularly used the withdrawal method for birth control. I knew that this wasn't ideal, but I had used it in the past and thought it would be okay. I guess I wasn't totally surprised when my period didn't come. I am not dumb. I knew the risks of what I was doing. Of course, the pregnancy test came back positive.

I knew I wasn't ready to have a baby. I was just figuring out where I was going to college and what I was going to do with my life. I made the decision to terminate the pregnancy, and while I am thankful that I had that choice, it was the hardest thing I have ever done.

—Casey, 33

Watch Out for Those Few Early Drops!

Before a man ejaculates, he releases a slippery, clear fluid designed to aid sperm survival and neutralize the acidity of the urethra through which the sperm travel. People often confuse these few drops of "leaking" with a man's inability to control his ejaculation. In reality, it is an absolutely healthy and necessary sexual function. But this pre-ejaculate, or precum, may contain live sperm capable of living inside a woman's body for about five days! So even rubbing against a girl's vulva, quickly "just putting it in," or using withdrawal can all lead to an unplanned pregnancy.

As you just read in the last vignette, it's a gamble, and a bad one, like leaving your car door unlocked with the key in the ignition in a dangerous neighborhood. Maybe the car will still be there, maybe not. You can always buy another car, but you can't turn back the clock. It's something that you just don't want to risk.

PROTECTING YOURSELF FROM SEXUALLY TRANSMITTED INFECTIONS (STIs)

(For more specific information, see Appendix D on page 163.)

You can contract an STI from sexual intercourse as well as from any other form of contact in which bodily fluids are exchanged (including oral sex, anal sex, and even just rubbing your vulva up against a penis). And since some STIs are incurable, can lead to infertility, and may even be fatal you should use your newfound smarts to be assertive when it comes to taking care of yourself.

> *I very much regret messing around with a guy that I wasn't seriously involved with. Now I have an STI for the rest of my life to remind me of this mistake.*
>
> —*Mary, 30*

I dated a few partners before I met my husband. When I was married and 6½ weeks pregnant, I got a horrible pain in my right side and was rushed to the hospital only to find out it was a tubal pregnancy and nothing could be done to save it. I was left with the pain of losing a baby and the astonishing news that I had contracted chlamydia, which had caused scar tissue to form in my tubes. Neither of us had any symptoms. In the end, I was truly one of the lucky ones because they were able to treat it and save my other tube.

I now have children and am truly thankful because I was told that chlamydia can lead to infertility if left untreated for too long. When I was young, I never thought that having only a few partners would lead to an STI or possibly even ruin my chances of ever having children.

—Lexie, 29

When I was 18, I was in a monogamous relationship with a sweet man who got a cold sore one week. It wasn't a big deal to either of us, and he avoided kissing me on the mouth. When it was no longer so visible, we had oral sex and didn't even think about the possibility of genital herpes transmission. But of course, it happened. I was devastated. He was horrified.

We always used condoms, I was on birth control, we were monogamous, and we'd been tested—in short, we didn't realize we were taking any real risks. But we had. The initial outbreak was profuse and painful. The stigma was unavoidable. It has meant having "the talk" with any new potential sexual partner, and risking embarrassment and rejection, but there's no going back since there's no cure.

—Nicole, 32

You should also be aware that the Pill and other hormonal contraceptives do *nothing* to protect you from STIs. In fact, the Pill can actually put you at greater risk for contracting human papillomavirus (HPV), which in turn can put you at greater risk of developing cervical cancer! Only a condom can reduce your risk of both unplanned pregnancies *and* STIs.

I got HPV at age 20. Stupid me thought that being on the Pill meant I was safe from STIs.

—Lynne, 42

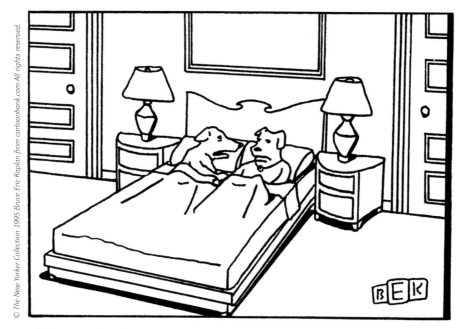

© The New Yorker Collection 1995 Bruce Eric Kaplan from cartoonbank.com All rights reserved.

"Since we're both being honest, I should tell you I have fleas."

A friend and I spent an evening with a couple of older guys who bought some alcohol. We drank with them at their apartment and things moved on from there. Later that evening, I ended up sleeping with one of them. He conveniently failed to tell me that he had herpes, so I contracted it at the age of 17. I was pretty sure that my life was over. Who would want to sleep with someone with a contagious, incurable disease?

In retrospect, it was probably a good thing that this happened to me. I realized that I wasn't headed in the right direction, changed my behavior, went to college, and became a much different person. And I made it a point to tell any man that I was involved with about the herpes. What was done to me was unfair; I wasn't going to do the same thing to someone else.

—Cassy, 33

Your Willingness to be Emotionally Vulnerable

Unless you are the Tin Man in *The Wizard of Oz,* it's pretty likely that you have a heart. That's a good thing, unless, of course, you value not getting hurt! One of the complexities of having sex is that it can touch your soul, in both magical as well as very painful ways. Still got that journal handy? Good. Part of deciding if you are ready to have sex is asking yourself some pretty tough questions, like:

* Will having sex decrease my self-esteem?
* How strong will I be if I end up feeling used?
* Will having sex end a good relationship or, maybe even worse, cause me to remain in a bad relationship?

When I was 19, I started to date a guy who was five years older. Our relationship turned out to be a rocky one, but I was desperately in love with him. He liked me and cared deeply for me, but was not interested in marrying me, which is what I wanted. We dated on and off again for 3 years.

A good friend of mine back then gave me some great advice—that good sex can make a bad relationship last longer than it should. She was so right! I knew that having sex was a very bonding experience, but no one told me while growing up that it would cause me to form such a deep emotional attachment to a person. It didn't seem to matter that the person was all wrong for me.

—Aria, 27

Another question you will want to ask yourself is how tolerant you are of double standards. As unfair as it is, your good reputation may be at stake.

All the boys I was around at age 13-18 were studs, popular and well-liked by each girl they "conquered." They rarely even liked the girl; they just had sex with her to win a bet or add to their score card. But the girls who had sex with even one boy were labeled a slut and harassed.

—Amy, 26

In the circles I ran in, it seemed being a virgin was the uncool thing to be, but the line was thin between that, and being a slut.

—Stephanie, 30

> *When I was 17, I had planned my first sexual experience with someone I knew and trusted well—my best friend. I felt that a lot of care went into the choice. The experience itself was more than a letdown, but even more devastating was the aftermath. Inevitably, even though we had promised each other not to tell anybody else about what we had done, the secret got out and circulated amongst our entire high school.*
>
> *Previously, I had a reputation as a very good student with great potential. Afterward, strangers knew a very private detail about me and used that information against me. I was looked down upon by peers as "easy" and "slutty."*
>
> *—Kate, 24*

Your Ability to Resist Pressure

When you just read the heading above, what did you think of? Maybe defending yourself from a guy who insists on having sex with you? Actually, *peer* pressure can be just as strong a factor in your having unwanted sex. In fact, that theme kept popping up over and over in the hundreds of experiences that women offered to contribute to this book.

> *At 17, many of my close girlfriends had already had sex. Lots of it. I felt like my virginity was a disease that I had to cure.*
>
> *—Ginger, 42*

> *My first time was . . . I don't even remember where it was! I do remember the boy. I was a junior, he a senior. We had dated for four or five months, and I thought I was ready. The truth was, all of my friends had done it, and I wanted to get it over with.*
>
> *In retrospect, I knew that my first time should have been more special, and I should remember it. I gave away the experience before I even knew what I was giving away.*
>
> *—Roxie, 32*

One of the most powerful things that you can do for yourself is to develop a healthy self-image. And that kind of confidence comes from knowing your body inside and out, developing special strengths and talents, and trusting in yourself to make choices that you will not regret in the future. By growing your confidence, you will be able to assert yourself in situations that may not feel right to you.

In fact, the kind of pressure that *individual* guys can put on you is something you should be prepared for way before it occurs. And one way of doing so is to internalize the following: Any guy who holds sex over your head as the key to his heart does not truly care for *your* heart (or your health). In short, you can and should resist this pressure with simple self-respect.

Just days after my 14th birthday, I agreed to sneak out of my parents' house with a girlfriend. One of her 21-year-old male friends was in the car and started paying a lot of attention to me. By the end of the night, I let him lead me behind a building. I was very nervous and scared and didn't know what to do, so I allowed him to have sex with me.

It was my first time and I was terrified, but I thought I had earned his love by having sex with him. I quickly learned that all I had earned was a broken heart and the loss of ever having a loving, wonderful, and meaningful first time.

—*Courtney, 28*

When I was 19, I was in college and hooked up with a guy I dated a little in high school. We hung out, cuddled together in bed, but I wasn't going to sleep with him. He tried everything to get me to give in, but gave up after he told me he loved me and I started to laugh, saying "No you don't!" He was shocked I said that, but he didn't deny it. I didn't sleep with him, but I did earn his respect.

—*Jenn, 35*

I was extremely self-conscious going into high school, so when I met an older guy who took an interest in me from another school, I was on Cloud Nine. I didn't want to give in, but I didn't want to lose him, either. I eventually did give in and hated myself for it. I would cry and pray at night for the strength to say no next time, but it never worked.

It still sickens me to think about how low I went to try and find self-worth. I'm so blessed to have made it through high school with no STI or unplanned pregnancy, and to now be married to a wonderful man.

—*Tina, 25*

Getting Real About Date Rape

Of all the types of unwanted sexual pressure, perhaps none is more harmful than those incidents that end up in date rape. One of the biggest misconceptions that people have is that you can only be raped by a stranger. Not true. Any situation in which you are forced to have intercourse against your will is considered rape, *even if you know the person, and even if you have had sex with them in the past.*

You should also know that date rape is considered any kind of sex you have with a date in which you are forced to do something against your will, whether or not you have been physical with this person before. No means NO, period.

If you have been the victim of date rape in the past, know that it is not your fault and there is nothing to be ashamed of. You can get help by calling the National Sexual Assault Hotline (1-800-656-HOPE; see page 173) or by talking to someone you trust to get support.

HOW TO STAY SAFE

Here are some things that you can do in the future to try to avoid this situation:

- Decide on your personal sexual limits *before* you go out, and communicate them clearly to your date.

- Be assertive, knowing that you have the right to protect your body.

- Know that you have the right to change your mind, even if you have started to be physical with a guy. Do not let him pressure you by claiming that he is in too much pain or will have "blue balls" if you don't have sex with him (he may be uncomfortable, but I promise you, he'll live).

- Avoid alcohol and drugs, which may impair your thoughts and actions, since some form of alcohol is very often involved in date rape. If you do choose to drink, don't let your drink out of your sight, since someone could slip a drug in it, which could compromise your ability to protect yourself. (The most common "date rape" drug is Rohypnol. This type of drug can make a person act without sexual inhibitions or even cause unconsciousness. You can learn more about it on the Internet.)

- Carry extra money or a cell phone with you so that you can get home or make a phone call for help.

- TRUST YOUR GUT: If something doesn't feel right, get out of the situation. If he doesn't understand, gets angry, or is demeaning, don't worry about hurting his feelings.

Your Expectations for the Relationship (Especially Your "First Time")

Part of deciding if you are ready for sex is to ask yourself what you want from a particular relationship. Is this someone you respect? Is this a guy you consider a friend first? Do you feel you can trust him? Regardless, the strongest relationships are often those that *don't* involve sex, because the couple has decided that they want to wait until they are married or until they know each other better, or because they don't want to ruin a great friendship by introducing the inevitable changes sex brings into a relationship.

Two of the greatest regrets women often discuss are with *whom* they chose to have sex for the first time and *when* they had it. Because your first sexual experience will undoubtedly be one of your most memorable life events, good or bad, these are issues that you may want to explore in your journal before you ever become sexually active.

> *My first lover was nice and considerate, but he was also young and inexperienced. He had no idea what to do to please me. Having sex, to me, was a major waste of time. I really don't think it is supposed to be like that. I was blasé about sex for a long, long time after that.*
>
> *I think younger girls really need to get in touch with themselves and demand to be treated right as early as possible. Celibacy is better than bad sex. Masturbating is much better than an abusive or careless boyfriend.*
>
> —Colleen, 42

> *I am 33 now, and was 16 when I lost my virginity to a boy who I had dated for about a year before we had sex. Up until the time we did it, we had mostly just fooled around a lot—but we had a very strong emotional connection. I would not have called it that when I was 16, but looking back, and comparing my story to what my friends' experiences were, I'd say we were much closer to each other than they were with their first partners.*
>
> *My experience was extremely positive. In fact, I often think in my day-to-day life how happy I am to have had such a good partner. He was patient; never pushed me; and we talked about—even fantasized together on the phone—what having sex with each other would be like. I was not his first, but he treated me like I was. We used a condom. And he asked me how I was feeling, worried I might be in pain.*
>
> *The act itself . . . not so great—it was awkward, a little goofy, and a little painful. But how we felt after . . . amazing. So close. I felt totally safe with him. I knew I made the right choice. We remained friends after breaking up about 7 months later, and continued to be friends past high school into our adult lives.*
>
> —Lisa, 33

Your Ability to Communicate Your Needs to Your Partner

Have you noticed the one theme that seems to come up over and over again in the women's stories you've been reading? It relates to the word I mentioned earlier that should always be at the center of every sexual decision: *respect*.

And once you have developed a respectful relationship with a guy, the most important thing you should both bring to the relationship is good communication. For some reason, it's human nature to assume that if two people are close, they should be able to read each other's minds, especially when it comes to sex. Wow, is *that* a wrong assumption!

In fact, the reverse is true: Those people with the best relationships will tell you that the most important quality that keeps their relationship so strong is their ability to be open with their partner about e-v-e-r-y-t-h-i-n-g. More specifically, if you think it will be awkward to *talk* about sex, you can pretty much assume that having sex won't be any easier!

This means expressing your needs and desires about how you want to be treated, and more generally when it comes to sex, what you like and don't like. It may sound unromantic to discuss these things, but the truth is that a relationship can only get better and better when you are able to be honest and trust each other.

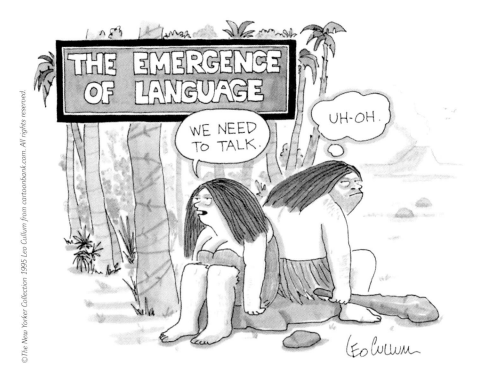

© The New Yorker Collection 1995 Leo Cullum from cartoonbank.com. All rights reserved.

When I was 18, I had my first serious boyfriend. He was funny and charming and smart, but for some reason, he got it in his head that all he had to do was put his tongue in my ear and I'd soon be "ready." Well, that's not how my ears or body worked, but even worse, he didn't have any idea what a clitoris was, much less where MINE was. Unfortunately, I never had the heart or courage to tell him how incompetent he was, and that's something I regret to this day. He was a good guy, and after he moved to another state, I'm sure someone more communicative made him a much better lover.

—Cathy, 27

I was "blessed" (for lack of a better word) because my first real relationship that included intercourse was not on top of a car or at a party. My boyfriend and I had our first experience in a planned atmosphere when I was 16 and he was 19. I was with someone who cared about me and my feelings. We had a fun relationship that lasted over two years. My experience with lovemaking in that situation made me realize that I did not have to sleep with many people to get satisfaction. What I DID want to do was be in a relationship with someone who cared about me and had respect for me as a person.

Respecting myself was number one—it was key. I was lucky . . . sometimes you seem to find the "perfect guy" and then find out he was totally NOT the person you expected him to be. In a way, we are all like that in the beginning of a relationship— hiding our faults, our shortcomings, etc. But to be in a relationship where two people genuinely want to get to know each other—ahhh—that is what makes it unique . . . and a bond.

—Ashley, 35

✳ SOME JUICY WORDS ABOUT UNDERSTANDING YOUR SEXUALITY

Sex, as you have been reading, can be the source of wonderful pleasure but also of serious concerns. And as mentioned earlier, one of the most important decisions you will probably ever make is with whom you have it and when you choose to do so. Hopefully these anecdotes have gotten you to start thinking about your own sexuality, and how it relates to all the remarkable things that you have previously learned about your body and cycles.

OK. Enough about all those yada-yada downers such as the risk of unplanned pregnancies and STIs. Despite the wide scope of subjects covered in this chapter, the "take home" piece can be summarized in four little words . . . four little words that can change your life. Commit them to memory, make them your mantra, own them. They will serve you again and again.

Knowledge: Good.
Ignorance: Bad.

Play them like a radio station in your head when you're at the crossroads of any important decision. Think of them as a radio station, "KGIB," constantly broadcasting in your ears.

And with that said, it's now onto the fun part of being a girl—your clitoris. This critical part of your anatomy is actually hidden from view, yet it is the center of sexual sensation. If it sounds important to find it, you're right. It is rich with sensitive nerves, and serves only one main purpose: to provide sexual pleasure.

So how do you find it? Start the treasure hunt at your belly button, and draw an imaginary line down toward your vagina. There you'll find it, below the line where your pubic hair starts, and above your urethra (otherwise known as the opening where you pee). It's under a hood of skin about an inch above your vaginal opening.

While exploring your vulva (what . . . you haven't taken out that mirror yet?) the really observant among you may have had an "Aha!" moment when you realized that your clitoris, the most sexually receptive part of your body, lies *outside* of your vagina, where sexual intercourse occurs. Given this, what follows should not be surprising.

Why Men and Women Experience Intercourse so Differently

For one thing, women don't achieve orgasms the way men do. They're simply not built the same way. A man's most wow-does-this-feel-incredible nerves are just below the tip of the penis, which is the part most stimulated during sexual intercourse, so men can achieve orgasm fairly easily. By contrast, as you now know, the most sensitive sexual nerves in *women* are in the clitoris, which is outside and above the vagina. So only about 30% of women achieve orgasms from intercourse alone.

> It wasn't until my senior year in college that I discovered what an orgasm was, and that's because I finally had a boyfriend who really knew anatomy! Besides being smart, he was sensitive and loving, and obsessed with what gave me pleasure. Too bad I didn't meet him sooner.
>
> —Susan, 28

I was 14 when I found myself with a boyfriend, and after a few months of fooling around we decided to "do it." I was sore, stinging, and bleeding, and very disappointed the first time. It was nothing like what I had expected!

For the next 10 years I continued to have sex with my boyfriends, looking for the sensations that I'd been led to believe were easily achieved by all women! It stopped hurting, but I never enjoyed it. Eventually I started to pretend to have orgasms so the boys wouldn't think there was something wrong with me. I was ashamed of my "disorder" and didn't tell anyone that I had been faking it every time.

—Marcy, 37

*After sleeping with a boy in high school for many months, it became clear that I enjoyed sex less than he did. He said there was something wrong with me because I couldn't have an orgasm through intercourse. In retrospect, now that I understand that women achieve orgasms differently than men, it makes me so angry that I believed **him** rather than myself in regard to my own body.*

—Kim, 34

Another major difference between the genders is that women are much more likely to view lovemaking as an emotional and intimate experience, and not just a physical act. And since a woman's physical experience of sex is quite different from a man's simply because her clitoris is located outside of her vagina, this little detail of location can have a dramatically BIG affect on every aspect of a woman's emotional and physical sexuality.

Throughout my teen years I had a tendency to have sex with any guy who desired me. Partly I was responding to the pleasure of being desired and partly I was under the mistaken impression that, as a newly liberated woman, I was required to have sex like a man—at every and any opportunity. The irony of this is that I never had an orgasm from any of these experiences. Only one of these casual partners ever, ever, ever inquired about my own pleasure. So, while I was sexually active (and always used birth control!), I acquired some very debasing and unfulfilling sexual habits that followed me into my marriage and greatly inhibited my ability to enjoy sex.

—Diana, 49

I remember my first time very well. I was a lot older than my peers before having sex and it became a sort of Catch-22. There was an upperclassman in college who was cute and we were kissing and things got heated. He wanted to take it further, but when I told him I was a virgin, he backed off, telling me this wasn't the right experience for my first time. I have to give the guy credit.

The thing was, it kept happening. I wasn't seeing anyone, but really felt behind the curve. Finally, one of my classmates agreed to, well, initiate me. He was nice and considerate, but it was over so fast. I remember thinking, Is this what all the fuss is about? *and feeling confused. So many magazine articles, movie scenes, and hushed discussions about sex, and the whole thing seemed way overrated. It wasn't until later, when I was in a long-term relationship with my boyfriend, that I came to appreciate how physically and emotionally powerful the act of intimacy could really be.*

—Sandy, 48

Finally, you may have already suspected that a woman's sexuality is often closely tied to her cycle, with many women tending to feel more sexual around ovulation. When you think about it, that certainly isn't surprising, since this is one powerful way to guarantee that the human race will continue to reproduce!

❋ COMING FULL CIRCLE: STAYING CYCLE SAVVY IF YOU'RE SEXUALLY ACTIVE

Now that you've had a chance to learn from so many other women's experiences, I trust that you will make the most enlightened decisions you can when it comes to sex and all of its potential pitfalls. If that means postponing intercourse until the right time and person, then great. But if you ultimately choose to be sexually active, using condoms is a non-negotiable no-brainer, at least until you are older and in a long-term monogamous relationship.

Although the Pill and other hormonal contraceptives are considerably more effective (see Appendix C), you can use condoms to both dramatically reduce the risk of STIs *and* have birth control failure rates that are nearly as low. How? Well, think about it. All contraceptives can fail, but they only fail when you are in that phase of your cycle when you are actually capable of getting pregnant—in the days approaching ovulation and immediately afterward.

You, of course, as the savvy reader that you are, now have a general understanding of when this occurs in your body. So if you do choose to have sex, protect yourself the smartest way possible.

If you are having sex, use a condom each and every time. Only condoms can protect you against STIs. And for those days in which you have wet cervical fluid or a wet vaginal sensation, you should try to double up your protection against unplanned pregnancies with an additional method, such as a spermicidal cream or the sponge. Better yet, if you were to postpone sex during those few wet-cervical-fluid days while using condoms the rest of your cycle, your risk of an unwanted pregnancy would drop dramatically.

If you think you may have gotten pregnant, regardless of the reason, you should be aware of emergency contraception, which will reduce your risk of an unplanned pregnancy by at least 75% if taken within 5 days of unprotected intercourse. See page 160.

A critical point before moving on: As well as you know your body and cycles, you can't assume that you could *ever* have unprotected sex without the risk of an unwanted pregnancy. Your current knowledge of Fertility Awareness is a wonderful foundation, but it does not give you the ability to "estimate" when you are safe during your cycle! The fact is that sperm can live up to five days or longer inside your body, and thus you simply cannot apply what you've learned in this book as a method of natural birth control! Also, I'll say it again: Fertility Awareness offers *no* protection from STIs. In case you were just distracted by munching on a cookie, let me repeat: **You simply *cannot* apply what you've learned in this book as a method of natural birth control!**

Fertility Awareness in Your Future

The truth is, there *is* a form of natural birth control that is based on the principles you've learned in this book. It's called the Fertility Awareness *Method*, (or FAM). However, such a method requires learning a series of fairly detailed rules and adhering to them *without exception*. It takes commitment to learn and stick to it, and yes, once again, it offers no protection from STIs!

Still, it can give older women a natural and empowering alternative to many of the other forms of contraception, which are often either a hassle to use or come with unpleasant side effects and physical risks. So it may be a great method for you to consider *in the future*, once your cycles are more regular, your life is somewhat predictable, and you are married or have a long-term monogamous partner who is willing to learn the method with you.

After reading the varied and often poignant experiences all these women had, what did you come away with? Again, the key theme that jumped out at me was how great sex could be, but at the right *time* and with the right *person!* Read on for a little more reinforcement of that idea.

I was brought up very strict Catholic—and that meant that sex was something that you only did with your husband and only to have children. When I was 16, I had, in my mom's mind, become a woman and we had "the sex talk." The one thing that she told me that has always stuck with me is to make sure that I was in love with someone before I considered sleeping with him. She didn't say to make sure you are married; she said make sure you are in love. She stressed that sex was something that two people shared as a deeper connection. Of course she did discourage me from having sex at my age.

When I was 17 and still a virgin, I was dating a guy who was 21 and also a virgin. We had a great relationship and were in love and lost our virginity to each other. I can honestly say that I had a wonderfully positive first experience with sex and that eventually led me to a wonderful marriage with another man. I consider myself to be very open about sex and will be with my daughter. And I thank my mom for allowing me to banish the negative views on sex and follow my heart.

—Jane, 34

I am one of those few "weird" people who waited until she got married to have sex, and therefore have had sex with only one man. There were times throughout high school that I was tempted—very tempted—but through one way or another, I waited for my husband. I cannot understand sharing that much of myself with someone I hardly know. Or even sharing it with someone whom I loved but didn't fully trust.

When we have sex, we are truly making love. We are showing an outward expression of the bond that we share. There is a moment when you are completely intertwined with this other person, and it feels like no one else has ever existed. It is just the two of you. You can see and feel the ultimate love he has for you, and he sees and feels the same thing in you. I don't know if you can experience it with more than one person. I don't want to find out.

—Kristi, 22

In my teen years I had such low self-esteem that I actually told a boy (in a roundabout way) that if he went out with me, I'd have sex with him. He still didn't go out with me, thank God! In fact, my first sexual experience was with a boy I liked. I didn't love him, but we were dating. It wasn't romantic, it hurt, and it pretty much killed my desire to have sex for a long time!

When I got to college I met my future husband. I was truly in love with him. Sex was wonderful, though it wasn't the fairy-tale kind of sex you dream about. But it was beautiful. I guess the lesson of my life is not to use sex as a bribe, or to have sex just because you're curious about it. Wait till you're truly in love and he's truly in love with you. It's one of the most intense things you can share with someone. Why would anyone (in hindsight) want to share something as intimate as that with someone they just like?

—*Valerie, 28*

My husband and I dated throughout high school and college, and married 10 years ago, when we were 21. Looking back at our dating years, I honestly have no regrets and I'm finding out more and more how unusual this is. We made a promise even before we officially started dating that we would not have sex. I can't say that promise was easy to keep.

We took every chance we could to be physically intimate. We enjoyed each other emotionally, mentally, and especially physically, yet without intercourse (it can be done!). My husband and I have a fabulous sex life now; it just keeps getting better and better. As hard as it was then not to give in to the social pressure to have sex, we stayed true to one another and we are so glad we did.

—*Liz, 31*

So there you go. Take the combined wisdom and experiences of all these women to heart. What they have shown you is that the decisions about whether to have sex, when to have it, and with whom are profound. To be sure, their most obvious message is that whatever choices you make, they should not be taken lightly, because the impact of your decisions will remain with you for the rest of your life.

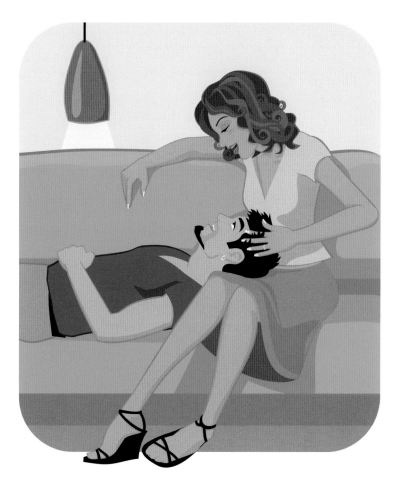

Of course, I think that every one of these women would agree that if you know your body well, you're more likely to treat it with the respect it deserves. For me, this might be one of the most important points of all, because respect for both yourself and your own body is exactly what being safe, cycle savvy, and sex smart is really all about.

Phew! This last chapter was pretty thought provoking, wasn't it? Why not find a quiet and private time away from all distractions, and take out that journal of yours. Try to answer some of these questions to help you make smart decisions for your life—decisions that you won't regret one day. This is a time to really reflect on what is most important to you. When answering them, be completely honest with yourself.

1. **What are my personal values and goals?**
What are my religious and political beliefs, needs and desires, educational and career goals, and future family aspirations?

2. **How would I react if I had an unplanned pregnancy?**
Would I tell my parents? Would I consider having an abortion, or would I give the baby up for adoption? Or would I consider keeping the baby? How would an unplanned pregnancy affect my goals and dreams for my future?

3. **Do I know how to protect myself from sexually transmitted infections?**
Do I fully understand that I could get STIs even if I don't have sexual intercourse?

4. **Do I get hurt easily?**
Do I care what others think of me? What would having sex do to my self-esteem? Do I get easily jealous?

5. **Am I strong enough to resist pressure, both from guys as well as my peer group?**
Do I feel the need to always do what my friends do in order to feel accepted? Would I consider having sex with a guy just so that he will stay with me?

6. **What are ways that I can take control to prevent date rape?**
Do I fully understand that one of the most effective things I can do to prevent getting into such a situation is to avoid alcohol?

7. **What are my expectations for relationships with guys (especially if I am having sex for the first time)?**
Do I want to wait until marriage to have sex for the first time? If not, do I want my first experience to be memorable? Do I want to date various guys, or only be in a monogamous relationship?

8. **Would I be able to communicate my needs to my partner so that I feel heard and respected?**
Would I be able to express my needs and desires without feeling awkward or embarrassed? Could I be assertive enough to say what I liked and didn't like physically?

Finally, you should internalize the answers to the following three questions:

* What is the one word that should always be at the center of any sexual decision you make?

* What is the only 100% effective way to prevent an unplanned pregnancy?

* What are the four little words that can change your life, and what is the acronym for the fictional radio station that can help you remember them?

seven

GROWING YOUR POWER AND CONFIDENCE

*h*ave you ever walked down a drugstore aisle and felt overwhelmed by the sheer number and variety of products designed just for women? By the looks of it, you would think that women's bodies were in constant need of being scrubbed down and sanitized from the inside out! Just look at the endless rows of douches, feminine hygiene sprays, deodorized tampons, and yeast infection medications, to name just a few. But are these products really necessary? Generally speaking, no.

For starters, your vagina is a model of hygienic efficiency, designed to clean itself in much the same way that tears act to keep your eyes clear if you get something in them. And as you now know, while it's true that you may occasionally develop a yeast or vaginal infection requiring treatment, the consistent pattern of cervical fluid that you see throughout your cycle is usually just your body's way of indicating that it is approaching ovulation. Being familiar with your own secretions will help you recognize the difference between normal fluids and actual infection.

So, rather than buying into manipulative douche commercials that only bring you down by implying that women are dirty, simply disregard them! You now know that just showering with mild soap and water will keep you clean and feminine. After all, women weren't designed to smell like a "summer breeze" or "field of white blossoms" as the feminine products would have you believe. The confidence that comes with understanding your body frees you to resist such hype.

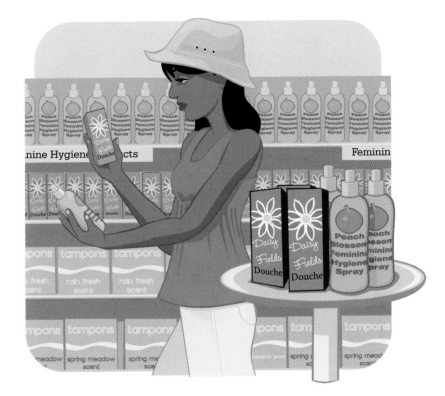

Even without all of the commercials that urge us to look perfect and smell like flowers, daily life can feel pretty overwhelming at times. Being a teenager, you probably have a zillion things happening at once. Between all your class projects, after-school activities, or the usual chaos with your friends, is it any wonder your life seems so hectic? To top it off, your body may mystify you if you don't understand what it is doing. When you add that to the other stresses of being a teenager, you have the perfect recipe for total crazy-making.

This is why, in so many ways, being intimately in tune with yourself is even more powerful than understanding history or math. But instead of answers being in a textbook, they are found in your own body. How practical is *that*?

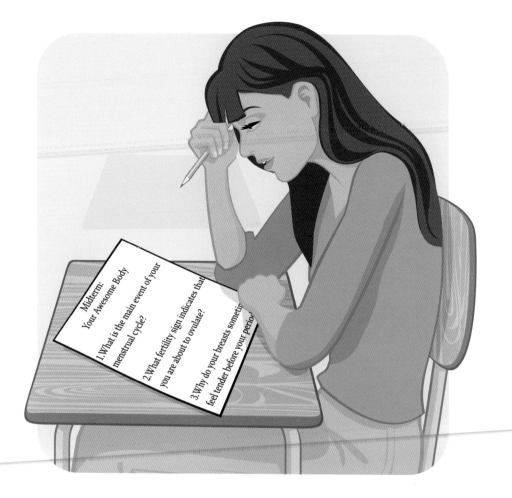

Midterm:
Your Awesome Body

1. What is the main event of your menstrual cycle?

2. What fertility sign indicates that you are about to ovulate?

3. Why do your breasts sometimes feel tender before your period?

With Fertility Awareness, your body is a wealth of fascinating information, and not a mysterious riddle that confuses you with "disgusting" or puzzling symptoms. Rather than worrying that you keep producing infectious "discharges," for example, you now know how to identify healthy cervical fluid.

In the last few chapters, you've learned that charting your cycle helps you see how amazing your body really is. The longer you observe your fertility signs, the more you will undoubtedly develop a sense of pride and wonder at the miracles it consistently performs. After all, it's hard not to be blown away by the fact that somehow, every cycle, your body knows how to accurately blend all the hormonal ingredients necessary for growing microscopic eggs—eggs that have the potential to develop from a few cells into a living, breathing human being in just nine months.

Admittedly, though, just being in awe of your remarkable body won't prevent you from experiencing some pretty embarrassing "female moments" now and then. Consider, for example, my own lovely experience:

I recently attended a concert in a beautiful hall downtown where everyone was wearing gorgeous outfits. During intermission, I ran to the ladies' room to change my pad. I was in such a hurry to get back that my used pad slipped out of my hands and landed within a couple inches of the trendy stiletto shoes of the woman in the stall next to me. I was so embarrassed that I tried to discreetly slide my dainty little hand under the stall to retrieve it. Needless to say, I waited until she left the bathroom before sheepishly coming out.

—Toni Weschler, your humble author!

By now you've probably noticed how easy it is for women to find themselves in awkward circumstances. But I bet you laughed when you read some of the blue-flowered vignettes like the one above, right? That's because the most embarrassing experiences we have are often the funniest when looking back on them. So wouldn't it be great if you had a sense of humor *while* you were enduring such distressing moments, just knowing that one day it would make a great story for your friends? So here's to a positive new attitude about surviving humiliation!

❋ UNLOCKING THE MYSTERY OF YOUR BODY: THE POWER OF BEING TRULY CYCLE SAVVY

Have you ever entered your house at night and freaked out because you feared the unknown? Of course, just turning on the light immediately reduced your fear, right? Your relationship with your body is similar. It can be incredibly illuminating to understand your body by charting. You can experience greater self-acceptance when you know how it works, because the mystery and anxiety usually vanish. This is especially true when dealing with those things that cause most women so much anxiety, from the "late" arrival of their periods to recurring breast lumps and other hormonal occurrences that they still haven't recognized as both normal and completely *cyclical*.

You may discover that in becoming an expert on Fertility Awareness, your own body is the first subject you have truly mastered! By learning such fundamental information about yourself now, you can avoid years of unnecessary worrying throughout the rest of your life. By charting, you'll soon learn your own body's baseline, and thus what's normal and not normal for you. In fact, you may know more about the practical realities of women's bodies than your peers, most adults, and even many doctors!

Fertility Awareness puts you, yourself, in the know. With daily charting, your cycle becomes essential to your life and sense of self, rather than just a dreaded monthly nuisance. Charting is an incredibly practical life skill that you are lucky to be learning at such a perfect age.

When you start charting your fertility signs, you realize that having knowledge about your cycles allows you a greater sense of personal control and empowerment that extends to all aspects of your life. In fact, your menstrual charts can easily become a type of permanent diary that allows you to keep track of everything, from particularly stressful events to special accomplishments. And of course, if you really know your body, you feel ownership over every aspect of your reproductive health, replacing ignorance with self-knowledge and expertise.

> *I have a friend who doesn't care at all about people knowing when she has her period. She holds her tampon up in the air on the way to the bathroom and doesn't try to hide it. It's really comfortable to be around her because she's not uncomfortable about it. When everyone else is embarrassed about it, it makes you embarrassed.*
>
> —*Ashley, 14*

❋ RESISTING THE PRESSURE TO BE PERFECT AND MAKING PEACE WITH YOURSELF IN A MANIPULATIVE WORLD

If you are like most girls, you probably can't get through the day without being bombarded with images of perfect models peering out of every magazine cover, or gorgeous actresses on television or in the movies.

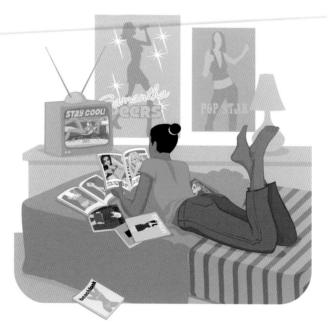

But do you realize that the majority of them are artificially enhanced in one way or another, either by airbrushing, tons of makeup, or plastic surgery? It's the nature of the business to make them appear perfect, even if it means resorting to flat-out deception! On top of that, many of these women spend hours and hours a day exercising, to say nothing of often starving themselves, all in an effort to achieve that virtually unattainable standard of beauty that 99% of us will never be able to reach.

One of the first and still most astounding examples of such deception that I can recall was a magazine cover from as far back as the mid-80s, in which the gorgeous model gazing out from the cover had flawless skin, huge clear eyes, and a slim and enticing body. Only one little detail escaped most viewers:

The model was not even a real human being!

She was a computer-generated image made to appear like the real thing, just like the gorgeous woman's face below, which—you guessed it—is also completely fabricated!

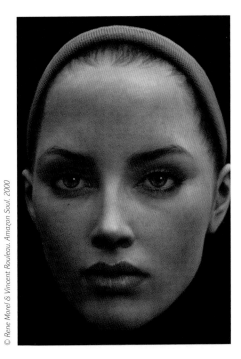

© Rene Morel & Vincent Rouleau. Amazon Soul. 2000

If magazine publishers can use nothing but a compilation of digital body parts to generate the appearance of a stunning real woman, you can be sure that most covers are touched up to eliminate any of the model's flaws. My hope is that once you realize this, you won't place such pressure on yourself to meet such a superficial and unrealistic goal.

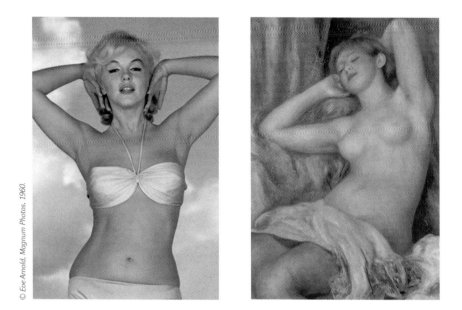

© Eve Arnold, Magnum Photos, 1960.

What do Marilyn Monroe and Renoir's beautiful nude above have in common? At another time or place, each one was considered the symbol of female perfection, even though by today's standards many would consider them overweight. Clearly, the perception of feminine beauty varies throughout different times and cultures.

As long as girls are filled with self-criticism, and as long as they're at war with their bodies, I don't know how we can instill in them a sense of wonder, curiosity, amazement, even awe about how their bodies work. The bottom line is something spiritual—viewing the body as a special, sacred vessel, to be treated with utmost care and love.

—Ms. Michal Schonbrun, Fertility Awareness Instructor

From what you've learned so far, you now know that your body performs some incredibly cool changes every cycle. Once you realize what a biological marvel you are on the inside, you can begin to appreciate how your outside appearance is only part of the package that is you. This is an important point, because we are taught in our culture to be dissatisfied with our bodies and looks. Fertility Awareness, however, helps us to respect ourselves, knowing we are complex and much deeper than the makeup and cute clothes that superficially define us.

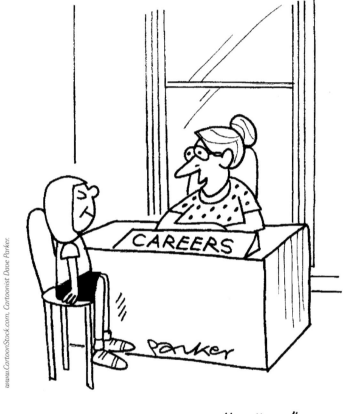

—BUT *APART* FROM 38" 22" 36" WHAT ELSE DO YOU WANT TO BE, CYNTHIA?

✳ THE PARADOX OF BEING BOTH UNIQUE
   AND COMPLETELY NORMAL AT THE SAME TIME

One of the interesting insights you'll probably have when charting is that your cycles make you both unique and completely normal simultaneously. In other words, your cycles are in many ways like a fingerprint. There are no two people on earth with exactly the same one. Similarly, no two girls will have exactly the same cyclical experiences. In fact, your patterns may be completely different from those of the girl who sits across from you in your geometry class. And while it's true that many girls will have somewhat regular 28-day cycles, some may have a fairly consistent 26-day cycle, while yours may vary between 27 and 32 days. The point is that they are all normal.

Some girls may find that they typically have only four days of bleeding and five days of eggwhite-quality cervical fluid, while others may discover that they tend to have six days of bleeding and only two days of eggwhite. And while you may notice that you tend to have a lot of breast tenderness the week before your period, your best friend may have an insatiable craving for salty foods for three days, but no breast tenderness whatsoever. See what I mean? Each girl is unique and absolutely normal at the same time.

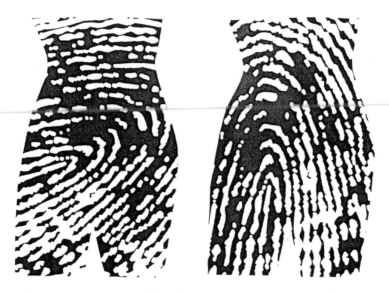

Lily usually has about a 25-day cycle, with four days of menstruation and five days of wet-quality cervical fluid. The second phase of her cycle is usually 13 days.

Mariah usually has about a 29-day cycle, with six days of menstruation and seven days of wet-quality cervical fluid. The second phase of her cycle is usually 15 days.

✳ HEALTHY, SAFE, AND SMART

Perhaps the last thing on your mind right now is your health, which you most likely just take for granted. You may be more focused on that English Lit paper that's due on Monday or even your prom at the end of the month. For the most part, teenagers can pretty much breeze through these years without having to worry about their health. (Dealing with strict parents or major crushes is another thing altogether!) In a weird way, maybe that's why it's at this time in your life that it seems so tempting to do things that will compromise that great health.

"Oh no, not again . . . here comes the lecture about no cigarettes, no drugs, no alcohol, no tattoos, no piercings . . . blah blah blah."

Actually, I'll spare you what you have already heard countless times before, since I trust that you are smart and probably get it by now anyway. I would just hope that by the time you finish this book, you will have gained such a profound respect for your body and how it works that you won't even be tempted to abuse it, which is what many of those things do.

And whether or not you have kids one day, the fact is that you will live the rest of your life in this incredible body of yours. Given this, wouldn't it be a great idea to become intimately acquainted with it, so you can forever treat it with the respect it deserves? Knowing your body well will allow you to make informed decisions about everything from what method of birth control will be right for you to what you can do to protect your future fertility. Note the key phrase here is "informed decision," an expression you will hear numerous times and in many different contexts over the years.

The bottom line is that you really can't make a good choice about anything unless you have all the facts about it. In the case of your own body, observing its cyclical changes on a daily basis provides you with basic information for making so many of life's most important gynecological and reproductive decisions.

✳ ENRICHING YOUR RELATIONSHIPS

Let's face it, cervical fluid is not the type of thing that comes up in casual conversation, even among best friends. Yet once you've learned to chart, you can dispense with whispers and embarrassment because you'll find it easier to talk to boyfriends, girlfriends, doctors, and maybe even your own mom about such things. One day you'll also be able to plan a family with your future husband with all the right information at hand, and most likely, educate him about you in the process.

Personally, I've always thought that one of the greatest benefits of learning Fertility Awareness is the way in which it can promote better relationships with those around you. Because the knowledge you gain is so practical, you will find that girls will probably come to you for answers to the most basic questions about their bodies.

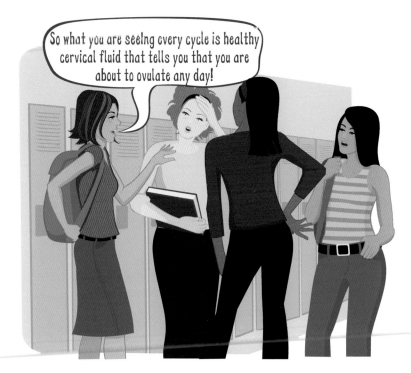

Being able to share this knowledge with other girls (and guys, in some cases) is a gratifying way to positively affect another's life. And because knowledge of Fertility Awareness can be passed down through the generations, you'll one day be able to help educate your own daughter (or even son!) in ways that will undoubtedly bring you closer to each other.

✳ EMPOWERING YOURSELF WHEN YOU ARE OLDER

With all you have on your plate right now, probably the last thing on your mind is deciding if and when you want to get pregnant. But a few years from now you will be among the first generation of women to be so knowledgeable about your fertility and cycles that you will be able to use the Fertility Awareness Method. As mentioned in the last chapter, FAM is a natural method of birth control and pregnancy achievement that allows you to accurately determine on a day-to-day basis when you can and cannot conceive.

So if you decide to learn FAM's specific rules in the future, you can read my book called *Taking Charge of Your Fertility*, which will help you manage your fertility without artificial hormones, other contraceptives, or medical intervention. And if later you do have problems getting pregnant (trust me—many before you did!), you will be way ahead of other women, because you will be able to help your doctor diagnose your problem early on and provide appropriate treatment most efficiently.

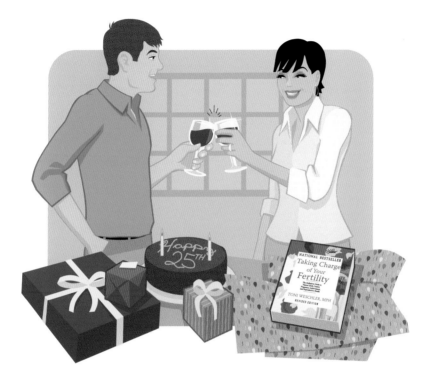

Ultimately, though, perhaps the most important benefits of Fertility Awareness and charting have little to do with everyday practicalities, but rather the sense of assurance you can have in finally knowing how and why your body works as it does. No, it isn't easy being a teenager, and it surely isn't easy being a female teen, but it's my sincere hope that by helping you finally unravel all those menstrual mysteries, you'll have a greater sense of pride in your own body. In so doing, you will undoubtedly grow into a healthy, confident, and cycle-savvy young woman.

The Art of Communication

Some intriguing questions for you and your mom

Are you embarrassed to talk to your mom about personal things? Try answering the questions below about yourself first. Then find a good time to ask your mom what her answers would be. Here's an excuse to finally open the door to great communication with her. Who knows—you may even discover that she's not all that dorky after all. In fact, you may just realize that she's actually pretty cool!

Questions	Me	Mom
How old were you when you got your first period?		
Did your mom have "The Period Talk" with you before you got it?		
How did you react to getting yours the first time? Do you mind having them now?		
Were they painful the first couple years? And now?		
Have you ever had an embarrassing experience with your period?		
Do you know when to expect it? If so, how long beforehand?		
How long are your cycles?		
Do you know when you ovulate?		
How many days of eggwhite did you have as a teen? And now?		
Did you ever go to the doctor because you thought your cervical fluid was an infection?		
What kind of secondary fertility signs do you experience?		
Did you know about Fertility Awareness when you were my age?		

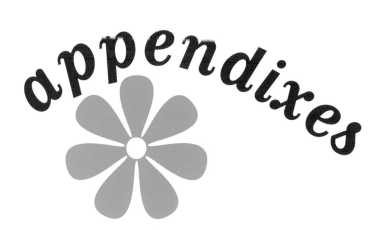

appendixes

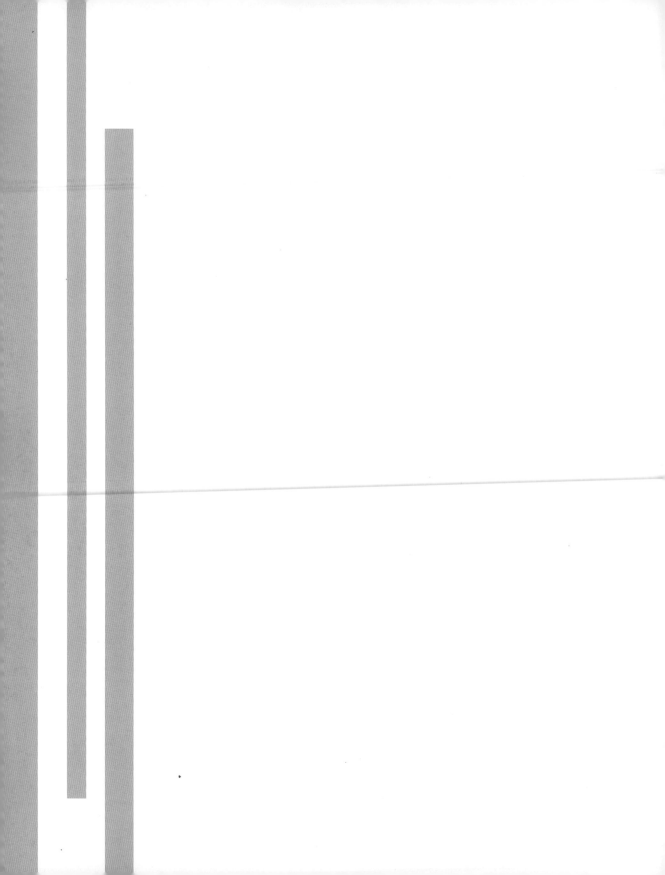

appendix a

THE LOWDOWN ON CHARTING AND THAT CLEVER LITTLE COVERLINE

This appendix is basically a short summary of everything you learned in Chapter 4 about observing and charting your two fertility signs. You can use it as a quick reference guide that you keep next to your charts. In addition, I included a couple of little temperature tricks that help make your charts even more understandable. One is called the Coverline (page 135) and the other is called the Rule of Thumb (page 136).

Have fun, and happy charting!

✳ WAKING TEMPERATURE

Taking Your Temperature

1. Take your temperature orally every morning, first thing upon awakening.
2. Take it about the same time every day.
3. Try to take your temps after you've had *at least three hours of consecutive sleep.*
4. Use an oral digital thermometer and wait until it beeps before removing it.

Charting Your Temperature

1. Record your waking temperature by circling the 1/10th degree above 97 or 98.
2. Record your temps with a pen, and everything else on your chart with a pencil. Omit the occasional outlying temp by drawing a dotted line between the normal temperatures on either side of it
3. Record unusual events such as stress, illness, moving, or travel in the "Notes" row at the bottom of the chart.

✳ THE COVERLINE: ADDING CLARITY TO CHARTING

A coverline is simply a line that you draw to separate the temperatures before ovulation from the temperatures after ovulation. Remember that the reason to chart your temperature is to determine when you ovulated in any given cycle. When you know that, you can then predict accurately when your period will be dropping in to say hello. No more panicked thoughts like "Uh-oh, I don't have any tampons and I'm in the middle of a tennis match . . . better fake a knee injury."

Remember that after ovulation, temperatures rise above the pattern of low temps you had before your egg was released. This temperature shift is often so obvious that you'll be able to spot it simply by glancing at the chart. However, a great way to see it more easily is by drawing a coverline.

When you first learn how to draw it, you may have a sneaking suspicion that I've pulled a fast one on you, and that this section really belongs in your math book. Actually, for many of you, you'll see right away how much fun it is. For others, it may take a few cycles before you get the hang of it, after which you may become the girl everyone else comes to for advice on how to draw their own coverline. Or not. But the point is that drawing it accurately should become fairly routine within a few cycles.

How to Draw the Coverline

1. A few days after your period ends, as you are charting your temperatures, always look back and keep an eye out for the highest of the *previous 6 days.* (So, for example, in Maya's chart below, imagine that she has been glancing back at the last 6 temperatures as her chart has been unfolding. On Day 20, in this example, she looks back at the last 6 days and notes the highest of those 6 temperatures—in this case, 97.6 on Day 17.)

2. As you continue along, identify the first day your temperature rises at least 2/10ths of a degree higher than that *highest* temperature in those preceding 6 temperatures. (In this case, 98.2 on Day 21 is at least 2/10ths higher than 97.6.)

3. Go back and highlight the last six temperatures before the rise. (In this case, highlight the 6 days before the rise on Day 21.)

4. **Draw the coverline 1/10th of a degree above the *highest* of that cluster of six highlighted days preceding the rise.** (In this case, 1/10th above 97.6 on Day 17, which puts the coverline at 97.7.)

5. Note that high temperatures during your period can be ignored when determining your coverline. It's not unusual to have high temperatures during menstruation due to the lingering effects of progesterone from the last cycle. Other outlying temperatures can also be discounted using the "Rule of Thumb" explained on the next page.

6. After drawing the coverline, you can count how many days are in the phase after ovulation by recording them from the first day your temperatures are above the coverline until the day before your period. (In Maya's chart below, Day 21 through Day 33 is a 13-day post-ovulatory phase.)

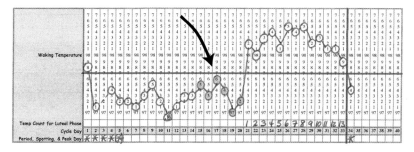

Maya's chart: She drew her coverline 1/10th of a degree above the highest of the preceding 6 temps before the rise on Day 21, making it 97.7.

Outlying Temperatures and the Rule of Thumb

If you have an occasional temperature that is artificially high due to reasons such as fever or a restless night's sleep, you may cover the outlying temperature with your thumb when you are determining your coverline. Hence, the "Rule of Thumb." Circle the outlying temperature as you would any other, but then draw dotted lines between the temperatures on either side, so that it doesn't interfere with your ability to interpret your chart. You essentially ignore the abnormal temperature, and thus still must count back the required *six* days, *not* including the day eliminated, to determine your coverline.

For example, in Nicky's chart below, Day 11 clearly shows an outlying temperature. So, she simply ignores it by drawing a dotted line between the Day 10 and Day 12 temps, and uses her thumb to cover the outlying temperature when interpreting her chart.

THE RULE OF THUMB

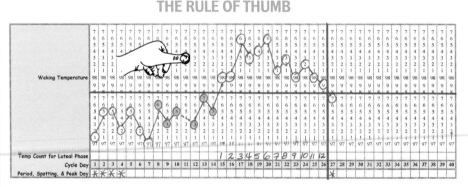

Nicky's chart: This cycle length is 26 days, since Nicky got her next period on Day 27. On Day 11, she noticed that her temperature was high and thought it might be her temperature shift. But the next day, it dropped back down, so she realized it was just an outlying temperature. So she handled it by drawing dotted lines on either side of it. Then, on Day 15, she thought that this may be the real temperature shift. This time, it continued to remain high, so she highlighted the six temperatures before the rise, and drew the coverline ¹/₁₀th of a degree above the highest (97.7), which in this cycle was 97.8. Finally, she counted 12 days in her luteal phase before she got her period.

Note that the outlying temperature during her six-day count did not prevent her from drawing the coverline. She merely passed over it by covering it with her thumb. You should also be aware that if there are a few consecutive days that are abnormally high because of something like a 3-day flu, then all of those temps would be skipped over when counting back 6 days.

✻ CERVICAL FLUID

Observing Your Cervical Fluid

1. Begin checking cervical fluid the first day after your period has ended.
2. Focus on vaginal *sensations* throughout the day.
3. Notice your underwear throughout the day.
4. Try to check cervical fluid every time you use the bathroom, at least three times a day, including morning and night.
5. *Before* urinating, separate your vaginal lips and use tissue to check your cervical fluid at the lower opening of your vagina, wiping from front to back.
6. Does your cervical fluid feel dry? Sticky? Creamy? Slippery?
7. Look at it and note the color, consistency, and amount.
8. Slowly open your fingers to see how much it stretches before it breaks.
9. *After* urinating, focus on how easily the toilet paper slides across your vaginal lips when you wipe. Does it feel dry, smooth, or lubricated?
10. Pay special attention to cervical fluid after a bowel movement.

Charting Your Cervical Fluid

1. Day 1 of the cycle is the first day of red menstrual bleeding.
2. Record what type of bleeding and cervical fluid you noticed during the day.
3. Record the most *fertile-* or *wet-*quality cervical fluid of the day.
4. Record the wettest vaginal sensation you notice throughout the day, since it is the most important indicator of where you are in your cycle.

CHARTING YOUR CERVICAL FLUID

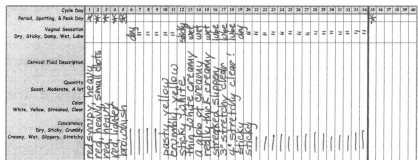

Olivia's chart: Olivia's cycle is 34 days because she got her next period on Day 35. She had a 5-day period, with spotting on the 5th day. She didn't notice any cervical fluid until Day 10, but even then her vaginal sensation felt dry or sticky for a couple more days. But on Day 13, she noticed that her cervical fluid started becoming wetter, and continued to be wet until Day 18. Notice that she had a very lubricative feeling on Days 16–18. The following day, it quickly dried up and she had a dry vaginal sensation through the end of her cycle on Day 34.

Identifying Your Peak Day

The last day that you produce slippery cervical fluid *or* have a lubricative vaginal sensation for any given cycle is called the "Peak Day," because it is your peak day of fertility. It most likely occurs either a day before you ovulate or on the day of ovulation itself.

You will only be able to determine the Peak Day after it happens, on the following day. This is because you can only recognize the Peak Day *after* your cervical fluid and vaginal sensation have already begun to dry up.

RECORDING YOUR PEAK DAY

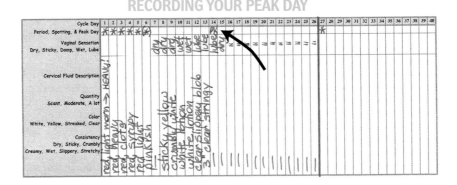

Peyton's chart: Peyton's cycle is 26 days because she got her next period on Day 27. She had a 6-day period, with spotting on the 6th day. She first noticed cervical fluid on Day 8, but even then her vaginal *sensation* felt dry or sticky until Day 10, when she noticed that her cervical fluid started becoming wetter, and continued to be wet until Day 13. BUT, notice that she had a very lubricative feeling on Day 14, even though she no longer saw any cervical fluid.

The following day, on Day 15, all the wetness dried up, so she was able to determine that her Peak Day was the day before, Day 14, the last day that she had a lubricative vaginal sensation. She marked that day with "PK" just above the "Vaginal Sensation" row. She had a dry vaginal sensation throughout the rest of her cycle, ending on Day 26.

appendix b

FREQUENTLY ASKED QUESTIONS

✻ OVULATION

✻ WAKING TEMPERATURES

✻ CERVICAL FLUID

❋ FERTILITY AND CYCLES

Is the first day of my cycle considered the first day of red bleeding or brown spotting?

The first day of red bleeding is considered the first day of your cycle. So you shouldn't start a new chart until you really start flowing.

How long can a human egg and sperm survive?

Most eggs probably survive about 6 to 12 hours, though they could survive up to 24 hours after ovulation. And sperm can survive up to five days inside a woman's reproductive tract, which is why you can't simply "guess" when you may or may not be fertile!

How does the Pill work?

The primary way that the Pill works is by suppressing ovulation. In addition, it prevents the uterine lining from producing a rich site for egg implantation, as well as prevents the cervical fluid from forming a wet, fertile quality necessary for sperm survival.

❋ GETTING PREGNANT

Is it possible to get pregnant even if I haven't started having periods yet?

Yes, since you always release an egg *before* you menstruate!

Can I get pregnant the first time I have sex?

ABSOLUTELY!

Can I get pregnant during my period?

Well, yes and no. Huh? The fact is that it's not possible to actually become pregnant during your period, but much more importantly, it *is* possible to get pregnant *from intercourse* during your period! In other words, since sperm can live for five days, a couple could have sex near the end of the woman's period, and the sperm could then live long enough to fertilize an egg several days later, if the woman had a very early ovulation.

Can I get pregnant at any time in my cycle?

No. It is true that ovulation can vary from cycle to cycle, but once a woman ovulates, she cannot ovulate again for the remainder of that cycle. But because of the risk of STIs, and because this book does not cover the intricate rules that identify exactly when you are safe from getting pregnant, you should consider yourself fertile every single day.

✳ BLEEDING

What causes very light or very heavy periods?

Exceptionally light or heavy periods can be the result of an anovulatory cycle—that is, a cycle in which an egg was not released. You can determine if you ovulated by whether you had a temperature shift 12 to 16 days before this type of period. If there wasn't a temperature shift, you can be fairly certain that the bleeding you are experiencing is anovulatory. Strictly speaking, this is not a true menstrual period, since it did not follow the release of an egg.

It is also important that you know the difference between anovulatory bleeding and ovulatory spotting. Anovulatory bleeding often feels like a real period. By contrast, ovulatory spotting is usually lighter brown or red, and usually occurs, as the name implies, about the time of ovulation. You can confirm that it was ovulatory by a temperature shift within a couple days of the spotting, followed by a true red flow within about two weeks.

If I have anovulatory bleeding, do I consider it a period and start a new chart?

Technically, a complete cycle goes from a true period to a true period. So charting anovulatory bleeding is a little different. There are two ways that you can handle it. If the bleeding occurs about the time you would expect a period, you will probably want to start a new chart, counting Day 1 as the first day of bleeding, even though you did not see a temperature shift about 12 to 16 days beforehand. That cycle is what is referred to as an anovulatory cycle, so the chart for it will clearly look different from the others. This is because it won't have an obvious temperature shift, and it's possible that the bleeding will seem different than normal.

The other option is to continue charting until you finally have a true menstrual period. In this case, you may end up having a really long cycle in which you have to tape together at least two charts. Of course, you will know when you have had a true menstrual period by the temperature shift that occurred about two weeks before the onset of bleeding. At that point, you can take out a clean chart and count your period as Day 1 of the new cycle.

What causes midcycle spotting?

About 10% of women will notice that they occasionally have a day or two of spotting about midcycle, right around ovulation. In fact, they may even notice that the fertile cervical fluid (especially the eggwhite quality) is tinged with brown, pink, or red. This is a result of spotting mixed with cervical fluid, and denotes an extremely fertile time. It is caused by the fluctuating hormones in the days surrounding ovulation.

❋ OVULATION

Do women always ovulate on Day 14 of their cycle?

No! The day of ovulation can vary among women as well as within each individual woman. However, once you ovulate, the time between ovulation and your menstruation is very consistent, almost always between 12 and 16 days. Within most individual women, this length of time generally doesn't change by more than a day or two. In other words, if there is going to be variation in the cycle, it is the first (preovulatory) phase that may vary. The second (postovulatory) phase generally remains constant.

Can a woman ovulate more than once per cycle?

No! Have you ever heard of a woman getting pregnant on Monday, and then again the following Friday, and then two weeks later on Thursday? Certainly not, because once a woman ovulates, her body cannot release any more eggs that cycle. Ovulation may take place over approximately 24 hours, but just once per cycle. During those 24 hours, one or more eggs may be released (as in the case of fraternal twins). But once ovulation has occurred, it is virtually impossible for a woman to release another egg until the next cycle.

Can you "feel" ovulation happen?

The most obvious outward sign of approaching ovulation is increasingly wet and slippery cervical fluid. In fact, it can be so abundant that you may notice a string of cervical fluid literally hang down when you use the toilet (yikes!). If you notice this, you should assume that ovulation is about to happen within a day or two. This is what is referred to as a primary fertility sign.

Some women are lucky enough to notice other signs on a regular basis, all of which are useful in helping them to further understand their cycles. These signs are referred to as secondary fertility signs, because they do not necessarily occur in all women or in every cycle in individual women. An example of a secondary fertility sign is the sharp pain that women often feel right around ovulation, which is called *mittelschmerz,* or literally, "middle pain." It is most likely caused by the egg bursting through the ovarian wall.

Do women feel more sexual around ovulation?

Many women do. Because estrogen peaks around ovulation, women typically experience a wet, slippery sensation due to the fertile cervical fluid they produce. This cervical fluid feels similar to sexual lubrication, and can therefore be experienced as a sexual sensation.

✸ WAKING TEMPERATURES

Do I have to wake up every day at the same time to take my temperature?

No, although you should try to be as consistent as possible. And even though you may sleep in on the weekends, most of you probably still wake up to pee every morning about the same time. In general, waking temperatures tend to creep up about two-tenths of a degree for every extra hour you sleep in. Thus, if you take it substantially later than usual, it may result in a reading that is outside your usual pattern. This is called an outlying temperature.

If you wake up earlier than usual, you should take your temperature upon awakening, so long as you have had at least three consecutive hours of sleep. Regardless, an occasional outlying temperature can easily be dealt with by following the Rule of Thumb (page 136).

What do I do if I missed taking a temperature?

No big deal. Simply connect the temperatures on either side of the missing day with a dotted line.

How do I handle taking temps on the weekends or when I sleep in?

You may be one of the lucky girls whose temperatures are not really affected by taking them later than normal. The way you will know is whether they seem higher than usual when you sleep in. If they are higher, than go ahead and still circle the temp, but do it only in pencil, and connect the temperatures on either side of the outlying temperatures with a dotted line. Better yet, even if you sleep in, you probably still get up to go to the bathroom about the same time every day. So just take it then before getting up.

How do I handle outlying temperatures?

If you have temperatures that are clearly out of line (for example, from fever, drinking alcohol the night before, or having slept in and taken your temperature late), just use the Rule of Thumb, covering any outlying temperatures with your thumb. Remember to draw a dotted line between the correct temperatures on either side of the outlying temperatures. In calculating the coverline, you count the six low temperatures before the rise, *not* including the outlying temperature (see page 136).

How do I handle erratic temperatures?

Some women may find that their temperatures do not seem to follow the classic pattern of lows and highs. For these women, consider trying any of the following:

1. If using a digital thermometer, verify that the battery is not low.
2. Consider trying a glass basal body thermometer, since digitals may be less accurate for some women.
3. If you do use a glass basal body thermometer, be sure to take your temperature for a full five minutes.
4. Regardless of which type of thermometer you use, consider taking your waking temperature vaginally rather than orally. (Of course, be consistent in how you take it throughout your cycle.)
5. Remember that certain factors can definitely increase waking temperatures, such as fever, drinking alcohol the night before, or not getting three consecutive hours of sleep.
6. Try to take your temperature about the same time every day. For every half hour that you sleep later than normal, your temperature may tend to creep up about a tenth of a degree. For every half hour that you wake up earlier than normal, it may tend to drop by about a tenth of a degree. You should note the time you take it in the appropriate column and use the Rule of Thumb to discount outlying temperatures that may result from sleeping late. (This will prevent you from mistaking a high temperature for a thermal shift before it has actually occurred. See page 136.)

How do I handle high temperatures during my period?

It is fairly common for women to experience several days of high temperatures during their period. This is usually the result of leftover progesterone from the last cycle or fluctuating hormones that occur during menstruation. Ignore the high temperatures during your period, and only connect those that are within the normal range. These early high temperatures will probably be above the coverline, but you can simply disregard them.

How do I handle a drop in temperature the day before my period?

Occasionally, you may notice an obvious drop in temperature the day before you get your period. While this is less common than when it occurs the first day of menstruation itself, it is still considered part of the luteal phase (this sudden premenstrual drop is caused by the disintegration of the corpus luteum). Day 1 of the new cycle is not determined by the day of the drop, but by the first day of bleeding.

How should I deal with charting my temperatures if I have a fever?

You will inevitably have a fever now and then. Yet this won't necessarily compromise your ability to understand your temperatures while charting, because your goal should be to identify a *pattern* of lows and highs, rather than focusing on individual temperatures. Assuming temps are off the chart, you can simply record the higher temperature above the 99°F, noting the fever and other symptoms of illness in the Notes row. Be sure to draw a dotted line between the normal temperatures on both sides of your fever.

Depending on the intensity of the fever and when it occurs, there are three possible impacts that it could have on your cycle:

1. It could have no effect.
2. It could delay ovulation (causing a longer-than-usual cycle).
3. It could suppress ovulation (causing an anovulatory cycle).

If the fever occurs after you've already ovulated, it almost certainly won't have an impact. If it occurs before you've ovulated, any of the three effects listed above are possible.

What does it mean if I don't have a temperature shift?

Now and then you may have an anovulatory cycle, meaning a cycle in which an egg is not released. If this occurs, you won't see a shift in temperatures from low to high because no progesterone will have been released to cause the temperatures to rise. Or you could be one of the small percentage of women whose bodies don't respond to the effects of progesterone, and therefore don't show a thermal shift even if you have ovulated.

What does it mean to have 18 or more consecutive temperatures above the coverline?

If you have 18 or more consecutive high temperatures above the coverline with no sign of a period, it is almost always an indication of pregnancy. The sustained high temperatures are due to the corpus luteum continuing to live and release progesterone beyond its typical 12- to 16-day life span.

Remember that most women will have a consistent luteal phase (the time from ovulation to menstruation). So, for example, if your own luteal phase is typically about 13 days, and your temperature remains high for 16 days, there is a good chance that you are pregnant. The point is to determine if the temperatures are staying high longer than what is normal for you. If you have had intercourse in the previous few weeks and your temps stay high for 18 days or longer, you should definitely see a clinician to determine if you are pregnant.

What does it mean to have a wet vaginal sensation or eggwhite-quality cervical fluid the day before my period?

Having a very wet, watery sensation or even an eggwhite-quality substance about a day or two before your period is absolutely normal. It is merely an indication that the corpus luteum has disintegrated, which it does before menstruation. The first part of the lining that typically flows out when progesterone drops is the water that composed part of the uterine lining. This watery substance should not be confused with fertile-quality cervical fluid.

What do I do if I have an infection masking my cervical fluid?

Vaginal infections produce many aggravations, including their ability to mask cervical fluid. What typically differentiates most infections from healthy cervical fluid is that infections usually have at least one of the following symptoms:

* ✳ Discharge, which is perhaps gray, green, foamy, or even like cottage cheese
* ✳ Itching or irritation such as stinging or burning
* ✳ An unpleasant or unusual odor
* ✳ Discoloration of the vagina, such as redness
* ✳ Potential swelling of the vagina and vaginal opening

If you realize that you have an infection, see a clinician for treatment. Record what symptoms you have and what medication you are taking, but understand that both will mask signs of healthy cervical fluid.

If you are sexually active, you should abstain from intercourse during this time in order to allow your body a chance to heal, and to prevent passing the infection back and forth between you and your partner. If nothing else, it can be extremely painful to have sex when you have one!

Why don't I ever have any dry days after my period ends?

Women who tend to ovulate fairly early, and therefore have shorter cycles, often start producing estrogen right after their periods end, so they begin producing cervical fluid early in the cycle. So noticing cervical fluid immediately after your period ends usually signals that you'll have an early ovulation with a short cycle.

What does it mean if I get patches of wet cervical fluid that come and go throughout my cycle?

Patches of cervical fluid that keep returning rather than going through the typical pattern of getting wet followed by drying up often occur in women who have either long or anovulatory cycles. In both cases, your body may attempt to ovulate several times before it finally does (in the case of long cycles) or may not ovulate at all even after several attempts (in the case of anovulatory cycles). In either case, the way to confirm if ovulation has actually occurred is to notice if you have had a temperature shift that has remained high for about 12 to 16 days before getting your period.

The one thing to watch for is if you have irregular cycles with this type of pattern. This could be an early indication of the condition called Polycystic Ovarian Syndrome (see page 29).

If my wet cervical fluid dries up, but I still have a lubricative vaginal sensation, which day do I call my Peak Day?

Great question! Your Peak Day is always considered the last day of *either* a wet-quality cervical fluid *or* wet vaginal sensation—whichever comes last. So, for example, in this pattern below, your Peak Day would be considered Friday, because even though you didn't observe any more wet cervical fluid, you still had a wet, lubricative vaginal sensation that day.

	Cervical Fluid	Vaginal sensation
Monday	Creamy	Wet
Tuesday	Creamy	Wet
Wednesday	Eggwhite	Wet
Thursday	Eggwhite	Lube
Friday	Nothing	Lube
Saturday	Nothing	Dry

appendix c

BIRTH CONTROL METHODS

It's pretty darn humbling when you think about it:

**The one and only purpose of your menstrual cycle
is to prepare for a potential pregnancy.**

That fact alone should be enough to convince you that if you are going to be sexually active, you must consistently protect yourself from an unplanned pregnancy, starting with the very first time you have sex.

There are a wide variety of contraceptives from which to choose, and while it's true that the hormonal ones such as the Pill and Depo-Provera are more effective in preventing pregnancy than the condom, the fact is that condoms are the *only* effective contraceptive that also dramatically reduces the risk of all those nasty infections.

The following pages contain a brief overview of the major contraceptive methods that are currently available, listed in approximate order of how appropriate they are for teenagers (alphabetized under each sub-heading). All entries are rated for both contraceptive efficacy as well as the protection they provide against STIs, which are the two most important factors in judging these options for teens such as yourself. The list concludes with a section on methods that are inappropriate for now, but are among the best for when you are older and married, or at least involved in a long-term monogamous relationship.

The listed effectiveness statistics show the typical failure rates for an average couple per year. The lower number is the *perfect* use failure rate (or method failure rate), meaning what percentage of women would become pregnant if the method were always used correctly over the course of a year. The higher number is the *typical* use failure rate, meaning what percentage of women actually get pregnant using that method over the course of a year. Obviously, many factors can influence these numbers, including the frequency of intercourse. But most importantly, the wide discrepancy often noted between the perfect and typical use failure rates shows that if you're going to have sex, you simply must use birth control methods *correctly*, each and every time!

An Example of Perfect Use Versus Typical Use Effectiveness Rates

If you and your partner always use condoms correctly, the chance of your becoming pregnant over the course of a year is about 2%. This is called the *perfect* use failure rate (or method failure rate) and again, it assumes correct and consistent usage each and every time. (To see what is considered correct usage and anything else you'd ever want to know about condoms, see pages 151 and 152.)

Unfortunately, there is often a big difference between the contraceptive *perfect* use failure rate and the *typical* use failure rate, which can be considerably higher depending on the method. For example, it's clear that many people do not use condoms correctly, and thus the typical use failure rate over the course of a year is closer to 15%, compared to the 2% perfect use failure rate. This means that for every 100 sexually active couples using condoms, about 15 women actually become pregnant. Obviously, the risk for any given woman will vary with the frequency of intercourse and motivation of the couple to avoid pregnancy.

What this means is that if you are sexually active and you make absolutely certain that your partner is using that condom correctly, you can reduce the risk to 2% per year. Still, even though correctly used condoms are very effective, they are not as effective as the various hormonal methods such as the Pill, which has an annual typical use failure rate of 5% and a perfect use failure rate that is well under 1%. But in addition to numerous side effects and health risks (see page 153), hormonal methods provide no protection from STIs, as in zero, zip, nada, not happening, no way, no how. So I do not recommend them unless, of course, you use them *in addition to* condoms.

❋ RECOMMENDED METHODS FOR TEENS

Abstinence

Effectiveness: Perfect. 0% failure rate.
Protection against STIs: A perfect 100%. (However, you should be aware that STIs can be spread through nonintercourse sexual activities, as well as through oral and anal sex! See page 163.)
Cost: Free.
Advantages: Natural, safe, no side effects, no problem! The absolute best way to avoid pregnancy, period.
Disadvantages: If you want to have sex, abstinence may not seem relevant to you (however, as discussed repeatedly in this book, you must then be responsible enough to choose another method to protect yourself, and use it each and every time).

Condoms

Effectiveness: Perfect use failure rate is 2% and typical use failure rate is 15%.
Protection Against STIs: Outside of abstinence, *the* absolute best method to protect yourself against the majority of diseases, including HIV/AIDS. Use them, use them, use them. *Every* time!
How they work: A tight-fitting sheath, usually made of rubber latex, polyurethane, or lambskin, is placed on the man's erect penis in order to prevent sperm from escaping into the female's vagina or near her vaginal lips. You can further increase their effectiveness by using them with a spermicide, as discussed on page 158.
Cost: Low (free to $1 a condom).
Advantages: Widely and easily available, many sizes and varieties for maximum sensitivity, and no side effects (although a few people are allergic to the latex from which most condoms are made).
Disadvantages: Can hurt spontaneity or mood of the moment, but they can also be a fun part of sexual play, if partners have the right attitude. Some guys claim they reduce pleasure (but there are ways around that; keep reading!).
Concerns: Lambskin condoms do not protect against some STIs, so it is better to use ones made of latex. To be effective against both pregnancy and STIs, condoms must be used correctly. If your partner is not experienced with condom use, it is up to you to make sure he learns.

The basics: Follow the instructions that are provided with the packaging, and always remember to:

* check the expiration date, and don't use condoms that are "expired."

* gently squeeze the condom wrapper in the middle to make sure it's filled with air (if it isn't, it probably has a hole in it and the condom should not be used).

* always store condoms in a dry cool place, and not more than a day or so in a guy's wallet.

* make sure your partner puts it on only after he has an erection, but before any genital contact or actual intercourse.

* make sure the condom is rolled all the way down the base of the penis.

* never allow your partner to stay inside you once he has ejaculated (if he gets soft before withdrawing, the condom could easily fall off and allow sperm to leak out).

* never use condoms with an oil-based lubricant such as Vaseline or baby oil, since these products can damage them!

* use latex or polyurethane condoms, but not lambskin (since the latter are not effective against STIs).

A final word on condoms and guys: Some guys will say anything to get out of using a condom, but I would say a boy who is willing to risk both pregnancy and STIs is probably not the type of person you should be sleeping with! Of course, the primary reason that guys want to avoid using them is that they think condoms make sex less enjoyable. In fact, there are now so many types of condoms that he should be able to find one that works for both of you, but regardless, here is a trick you can impress him with that may well change his mind on condom use:

Put a small amount of a water-based lubricant like K-Y or Astroglide on the glans of his penis (the underside of the head) just before putting on the condom. Don't use anything like oils or lotions, since they can break down the latex in condoms. For many guys, using lubricant will dramatically increase sensitivity, and thus, of course, greatly reduce his resistance to future condom use!

❋ HORMONAL METHODS

These are extremely effective contraceptives, but they offer *zero* protection against STIs. Therefore, it is highly recommended that if you use them, you do so only in combination with a male or female condom, each and every time! You should also be warned that one hormonal method in particular, Depo-Provera, below, is considered unhealthy for teenagers and probably should be avoided.

Depo-Provera

Effectiveness: Extremely high (only a 0.3% failure rate).
Protection against STIs: None.
How it works: This is an injection of hormones that prevents ovulation for three months. After that time, you must get another shot.
Cost: Around $30–$50 per shot, plus the cost of an office visit to a doctor or clinic.
Advantages: Easy to use, doesn't interfere with sex, no need to take a daily pill, and may decrease or stop menstrual periods (see Disadvantages below).
Disadvantages: It may stop menstrual periods, which could be very unhealthy for the female body to experience. Other possible side effects include headaches, mood changes, weight gain, abdominal pain, bloating, nausea, hot flashes, vaginal dryness, and sore breasts.
Concerns: It may cause bone loss in teenagers, so in essence, young girls develop old women's bones, putting them at increased risk for osteoporosis. And it can negatively impact blood cholesterol. Other side effects, such as weight gain, may take up to a year to disappear after getting the last injection.

Implanon

(This is a new method that has only recently become available in the United States.)
Effectiveness: Extremely high (extensive long-term studies have yet to be concluded, but it is expected that the failure rate will be as low as .05%, which would make it the most effective method available outside of abstinence).
Protection against STIs: None.
How it works: A thin tube is inserted just under the skin on the upper arm. The tube slowly time-releases a synthetic hormone that prevents ovulation.
Cost: Several hundred dollars, including an office visit.
Advantages: Easy to use, doesn't interfere with sex, no need to take a daily pill, and may decrease or stop menstrual periods (see Disadvantages below). The tube lasts up to three years, and can easily be removed at any time.
Disadvantages: It may stop menstrual periods, which could be very unhealthy for the female body to experience. Possible side effects include headaches, mood changes, nausea, weight gain, and sore breasts. The actual insertion of the tube can be a bit uncomfortable and can lead to some minor bruising or swelling for a few days. See "Concerns" above.

NuvaRing

Effectiveness: Very effective (a 1–8% failure rate).

Protection against STIs: None.

How it works: A small plastic ring is inserted deep into the vagina by the cervix, where it stays for three weeks before it is removed. After a seven-day break, a new ring is inserted. The ring releases estrogen and progesterone, preventing ovulation as well as decreasing wet cervical fluid and making it inhospitable to sperm.

Cost: About $10 per month for a new a ring.

Advantages: Easy to use, doesn't interfere with sex, no need to take a daily pill, and may decrease or stop menstrual periods. See disadvantages below. It can be easily removed at any time.

Disadvantages: It may stop menstrual periods, which could be very unhealthy for the female body to experience. Minor side effects may include headache, vaginal irritation or infection, nausea, and a change in vision.

Concerns: It may slip out! Certain women, including those who smoke, may be at increased risk for blood clots, heart attack, and stroke.

"The Patch" (Ortho Evra)

Effectiveness: Very effective (a 2–8% failure rate).

Protection against STIs: None.

How it works: A thin beige patch is applied to the skin on either the butt, abdomen, outer arm, or upper torso. It is replaced with a new patch once a week for three weeks, with the fourth week being patch free. It releases hormones that prevent ovulation, as well as decreasing wet cervical fluid and making it inhospitable to sperm.

Cost: About $10–$20 for three patches, or a month's supply.

Advantages: Easy to use, doesn't interfere with sex, no need to take a daily pill, and may decrease or stop menstrual periods. See disadvantages below. After it is applied to your skin, you can usually shower, bathe, and swim like normal. It can be easily removed at any time.

Disadvantages: It may stop menstrual periods, which could be very unhealthy for the female body to experience. Possible skin irritation at the patch site as well as other minor side effects, including nausea, tender breasts, abdominal pain, and menstrual cramps.

Concerns: It can become detached and fall off! Certain women, including those who smoke, may run a greater risk of blood clots, heart attack, and stroke.

The Pill

Effectiveness: Extremely high, assuming you remember to take it every day (a 0.3–8% failure rate).

Protection against STIs: None.

How it works: The Pill comes in a one-month supply of 21 or 28 pills that are taken every day (when taking the 21-day version, there is one week off before the next cycle of pills is begun). Most birth control pills contain estrogen and progestin (a synthetic progesterone), which prevent the ovaries from ovulating. There is also a progestin-only pill that allows ovulation, but prevents pregnancy by decreasing wet cervical fluid around the cervix in order to block sperm. It also inhibits the egg's journey down the fallopian tubes. This type of pill also makes the uterine wall inhospitable to implantation were a pregnancy to occur.

Cost: Usually about $10–$20 per month (clinics usually charge less than what it costs at a doctor's office).

Advantages: Easy to use, doesn't interfere with sex, may reduce menstrual cramping and frequency of periods. It may also reduce the risk of ovarian cancer and pelvic inflammatory disease (PID).

Disadvantages: Depending on the type of pill, you may experience side effects such as nausea, bloating, spotting, weight gain, breast tenderness, and mood changes.

Concerns: It's a lot easier than you think to forget taking the Pill, and the result of that, of course, is greatly increasing the failure rate of the method. Some girls, especially those who smoke (but why on earth would you smoke?!) are also at increased risk of blood clots, heart attack, and stroke. Increases the risk of cervical cancer if you already have HPV.

Pills Designed to Eliminate Periods

There are a number of new pills available that were specifically developed to reduce the number of periods you experience in a year, or eliminate them completely. While it may be very tempting to consider taking them, you should be aware that, as of this publication, there have been no long term studies to confirm their safety. In addition, there are many who believe that they can be *very* unhealthy for teens to take, especially since they seem to prevent girls from developing healthy bones.

You should also be aware that if you are sexually active, they will prevent you from knowing if you have had an unplanned pregnancy, because you will not have the benefit of your period or the withdrawal bleeding of traditional pills to indicate that you aren't pregnant.

❋ SOME OTHER METHODS

Diaphragm

Effectiveness: Medium (a 6–16% failure rate).
Protection against STIs: Some limited protection against some diseases (but not against HIV/AIDS, among others).
How it works: The diaphragm is a round, soft rubber dome that is inserted into the vagina and placed snugly against the cervix before sex. It thus blocks sperm from getting past the cervix, but to be effective, it must be used with a spermicide and kept in place for at least six hours following intercourse.
Cost: About $15–$25 for the diaphragm itself, an additional few dollars for a tube of spermicide, and the cost of an office visit to get the diaphragm fitted.
Advantages: Simple to use, rarely any side effects, and relatively cheap, since the diaphragm itself should last for years.
Disadvantages: For some women, it may be uncomfortable to insert, and it can be messy. A few people are allergic to the latex rubber it's made of, or to the spermicides that are used with it.
Concerns: It may increase the risk of urinary tract infections (although it may also reduce the risk of certain cervical STIs; life is tradeoffs!).

Female Condom

Effectiveness: Medium. Note that perfect use failure rate is considerably higher than the male condom (a 5–21% failure rate).
Protection Against STIs: Effective against most STIs.
How it works: A polyurethane sheath or pouch is gently put into the vagina before intercourse. There is a flexible ring at each end of the device that allows for the penis to be inserted, thus preventing sperm from entering the female's body.
Cost: Higher than a male condom (perhaps $2–$3 for each one).
Advantages: Gives you more control so that you don't have to depend on a partner to use a male condom. Easily available at drugstores. Can be inserted into the vagina up to eight hours before intercourse.
Disadvantages: Can be awkward-looking for both partners and may feel somewhat strange when being inserted.

IUD

Effectiveness: Very effective (a 1–3% failure rate).

Protection against STIs: None.

How it works: The IUD, or intrauterine device, is a small plastic object shaped like the letter *T*, with a short string attached to it. It is inserted through the cervix and into the uterus by a doctor or trained clinician, where it can remain for 5 to 10 years, depending on which type of IUD is inserted. It prevents sperm from reaching the fallopian tubes, and in addition, if fertilization were to occur, it prevents the fertilized egg from implanting into the uterine wall, thereby preventing a pregnancy.

Cost: Often $500 or more, which includes the cost of a doctor's visit.

Advantages: Once inserted, it will not interfere with sex. It can be removed easily by a doctor.

Disadvantages: Can increase the risk of pelvic inflammatory disease (PID), which can lead to infertility. The IUD can lead to heavy periods or cramping and occasionally chills and abdominal pain. It can also be very uncomfortable when the doctor places it inside the uterus (and on rare occasions the uterus may be perforated in the process).

Concerns: It may slip out of place, which is why the string should be checked every month. You should see a doctor if you have serious side effects or if you can feel the IUD with your fingertips protruding through the cervix. Not recommended for women with more than one partner because it places them at greater risk for PID.

Spermicides

Effectiveness: When used alone, not very effective (a 15–29% failure rate).
Protection against STIs: Some, against certain diseases such as PID (pelvic inflammatory disease).
How they work: Spermicides are chemicals that are inserted into the vagina before intercourse. They come in various forms, including foams, creams, jellies, vaginal inserts, transparent film, and vaginal suppositories. The chemicals are designed to kill sperm on contact. They are more effective when used in combination with condoms.
Cost: From $5–$20, depending on the type and amount that is bought (a tube that is enough for many acts of intercourse might cost $10 at a drugstore).
Advantages: Widely available in many brands and forms. Few if any side effects.
Disadvantages: Can be messy and may interfere with the mood of the moment. Occasionally, a person is allergic to certain brands or types that can cause irritation to the vaginal lining. This may increase the risk of getting an STI.
Concerns: Since the contraceptive effectiveness of spermicides is relatively low, it is advised that they be used only in combination with other methods, most obviously a condom. Be aware that only products with the words *spermicide* or *nonoxynol-9* on the label are genuine spermicides that protect you against pregnancy.

The Today Sponge

Effectiveness: Medium (a 9–16% failure rate).
Protection against STIs: Possibly protective against some types of STIs, but may actually increase the risk of HIV transmission. This is because the spermicide in it can cause some vaginal irritation, making it easier for HIV to be contracted.
How it works: The Sponge is made of a soft, disposable, non-abrasive polyurethane foam containing 1 gram of the spermicide nonoxynol-9. It is shaped like a half-dome that can be easily inserted into the vagina and placed over the cervix. It has a loop attached for easy removal. It works as both a barrier and a spermicide, but it is more effective when used in combination with condoms.
Cost: About $3 per sponge.
Advantages: A nonhormonal contraceptive that is immediate and reversible. Very comfortable and can be purchased without a prescription. Not messy.
Disadvantages: You cannot use it if you have an abnormal Pap test, genital lesions, infections, or if you're allergic to spermicide. May irriate vaginal lining if used more than once a day. There is a small risk of toxic shock syndrome (TSS), a dangerous condition caused by bacterial infection.

Withdrawal

Effectiveness: Not great (a 4–19% failure rate), but better than nothing.

Protection against STIs: None.

How it works: The guy pulls out of the vagina before ejaculation.

Cost: Free.

Advantages: No side effects. Can be used anytime.

Disadvantages: It can certainly interfere with the mood of the moment. More importantly, it makes you completely dependent on your partner's self-discipline to actually pull out before he has an orgasm, which is, to say the least, not a good idea. The bottom line is that this method is not recommended. Having said that, though, it is better than nothing if you find yourself foolishly using no other contraceptive method.

Concerns: Be aware that even if your partner pulls out with perfect discipline each and every time, the perfect use failure rate will not fall below 4% because men produce several drops of semen containing sperm that leak out before they have an orgasm.

✳ EMERGENCY CONTRACEPTION

The Morning-After Pill, or Plan B

Note that this is not a method of contraception, but an emergency backup that greatly reduces the risk of pregnancy if unprotected sex has already occurred, or if it is known that the contraceptive method that was used may have failed. It is, in fact, a very powerful drug, and thus you should be doing everything possible to make sure that you will never need it.

Effectiveness: A 2–24% failure rate, with effectiveness higher the sooner you take it after unprotected sex.

Protection against STIs: None.

How it works: Two pills are taken as soon as possible after intercourse, but no later than five days afterward. The pills are a very high dose of hormones that keep the egg from being fertilized by the sperm, or if that fails, that make the endometrial lining of the uterus inhospitable to a fertilized egg.

Cost: Varies widely, from free to $50, depending on where you get the pills.

Advantages: A good emergency backup for those who think they run a high risk of pregnancy due to careless behavior, ineffective contraceptives such as a broken condom, or even rape. For virtually all women, there are no significant medical risks. Available at some pharmacies.

Disadvantages: Common side effects include nausea, vomiting, bloated feeling, tender breasts, and mood changes. In some places, it must be obtained from a doctor's office or clinic.

A special note: If you do not get your period within three weeks of taking the pills, you should get a pregnancy test. Also, the morning-after pill should not be confused with the drug RU-486 (sometimes called Milepristone), which is used to cause a chemically induced abortion several weeks into a pregnancy. For more information on resources near you, check online at www.not-2-late.com to locate a health care provider or pharmacy near you that carries EC pills, or call the Emergency Contraceptive Hotline at 1-888-NOT2LATE (1-800-584-9911).

❋ METHODS FOR WHEN YOU ARE OLDER

The last three methods on this list are all different from one another in many ways, but they have two fundamental things in common: They are excellent forms of birth control, and yet they are simply not appropriate for you at this time in your life. Teenage girls such as yourself may already be physically and emotionally mature young women, but you still have colleges and careers to navigate, as well as fundamental decisions about potential partners and children. In other words, you still have a whole lot of living to do before you would find it appropriate to use any of the contraceptive methods listed here, so ultimately, they make sense only if you've already settled down with a significant or true life partner.

Fertility Awareness Method (FAM)

This is the natural form of birth control that is taught in my book *Taking Charge of Your Fertility*. It is based on adhering to four specific rules, all of which are grounded in the biological information you learned earlier in this book. Although FAM is an inappropriate method for teens, it should be easy to learn when you are older, since you will already be well versed in basic menstrual biology.

Effectiveness: Highly effective if the rules are carefully followed, and highly unforgiving if not (a failure rate of 2–25%).

Protection against STIs: None.

How it works: Women learn to chart their cycles, just as you have done in this book. With their charts as a foundation, they learn four very specific and detailed rules that allow them to know when they are considered fertile and when they are considered infertile on any given day. The rules take into account that sperm can live up to five days or longer, resulting in a fertile phase of about 8 to10 days per cycle. During this time, the couple can either postpone intercourse or use barrier contraceptives.

Cost: Virtually free (outside the cost of a thermometer and book or class to learn it).

Advantages: When used correctly, FAM is highly effective, and of course, it is natural and has no side effects. Perhaps most importantly, it is an excellent way for a woman to learn about her own body and keep track of her overall health. In addition, the information can be used to maximize the odds of quickly becoming pregnant when that becomes her goal. And finally, charting encourages male involvement, which draws many couples closer together.

Disadvantages: It may require a class or several hours of reading to truly learn the rules (which again, are not taught in this book!), and then several cycles or more to really understand how they are applied. The rules themselves must be very strictly followed, which means that the average female must either abstain for about 8 to 10 days per cycle or use a barrier method during that fertile phase. Finally, and as you already know, the process of charting can take up to a couple minutes a day.

A final comment on FAM: In looking at the disadvantages of this method, it's clear that FAM is certainly not a method for everyone, and given its lack of protection against STIs, it should be equally obvious that it will be appropriate for you only when you are older and involved in a long-term monogamous relationship. Having said that, though, I think it is an extraordinary way to both practice effective birth control and continuously learn about your body and cycle. I would therefore encourage you to explore it in the future, particularly if you enjoy the charting that you have already learned in this book.

Tubal Ligation

Effectiveness: Extremely high (a failure rate of less than 1%).
Protection against STIs: None.
How it works: This is the female equivalent of a vasectomy. In this case, an operation is performed in which the fallopian tubes are tied, cut, or cauterized so that the sperm are blocked from traveling to the egg, and the egg is blocked from traveling on to the uterus.
Cost: About $1,000–$2,500, depending on the doctor or clinic doing it.
Advantages: Permanent and hassle-free once it is performed. Although this operation is a bit more complicated than a vasectomy, it is still a relatively simple and risk-free procedure in which the woman is usually in and out of the doctor's office or clinic within a few hours.
Disadvantages: Like a vasectomy, it may cause some temporary soreness. In addition, while studies show that the tubes can be successfully reopened about 90% of the time, it is a costly and delicate procedure. Obviously, like the vasectomy, this is a method only for a couple that is sure they don't want any more children than they already have.

Vasectomy

Effectiveness: Extremely high (a failure rate of less than 1%).
Protection against STIs: None.
How it works: The man undergoes a simple surgical procedure in which the tubes that carry sperm between the testicles and the penis (called the vas deferens) are cut, so sperm cannot get through.
Cost: About $500–$1,000, depending on the doctor or clinic doing the procedure.
Advantages: Permanent and hassle-free once it is performed. The actual operation is short and simple (usually less than half an hour), so this is an outpatient procedure in which the man is usually out of the clinic or doctor's office in less than a few hours.
Disadvantages: The man may feel sore for the first few days after the operation. Most importantly, a more complicated operation called a vasovasectomy, which has only a 75% success rate, would be needed to restore male fertility. Obviously, a vasectomy is a method only for a couple that is sure they don't want anymore children than they already have.

appendix d

THE NASTY WORLD OF SEXUALLY TRANSMITTED INFECTIONS (STIs)

STIs are so named precisely because they are a varied group of contagious infections that are transmitted from one person to another through sexual contact. A couple of them have no known cure and can even been deadly. Many of them have annoying and even painful symptoms, some increase the risk of other infections, and others can cause infertility. Several can only be managed but never truly eliminated, and generally speaking, they are harmful to both your physical and emotional health. Other than that, they're no problem!

If you read the disease descriptions that follow, you'll quickly understand why postponing sex is a smart thing to do. Of course, if you are already sexually active, correctly using condoms is a no-brainer until you are older and in a trusting, long-term, monogamous relationship. Perhaps you don't want to keep hearing that, but trust me, as someone who has worked in a women's clinic, I can tell you from experience that you don't want to get one.

Here are a few key facts about STIs that you should know:

* You or your partner could have an STI and not even know it, since often there are no symptoms or they may have already disappeared. Be aware that just because a person has no symptoms does not mean they are not contagious. They still may have the actual virus, bacteria, or other source of the disease inside of them!

* If you have an STI, it's important to have your sexual partner(s) tested and treated in order to prevent further spread of the disease.

* Most STIs are detected by simple tests, and most can be cured with proper medical treatment, especially if treated early.

* STIs are spread through all types of sexual contact, including standard vaginal intercourse, oral sex, anal sex, and other sexual acts in which bodily fluids are exchanged between partners.

* There is a wide variety of STIs with all kinds of nasty symptoms and consequences (details in overview below), but generally speaking, you should be on the alert for the following possible warning signs:
    - Unusual vaginal discharge (including itching, redness, and an unpleasant odor)
    - Sores, bumps, or blisters near your genitals, anus, or mouth
    - Pelvic or abdominal pain
    - Unexplained fever

If you have any of these symptoms, you should see a clinician to have them checked, and avoid sexual contact until you get an accurate diagnosis and treatment. If you have an STI, you will also be asked to notify all sexual partners that you could have infected, so that they can also get proper medical treatment.

At a minimum, I trust that you will be sex smart, and that includes knowing what sexually transmitted infections are and how best to avoid them. I hope that if you do become sexually active, you will at least internalize the information in this overview, and based on what you learn here and from other sources, that you will always make intelligent decisions that protect the physical and emotional health of you and your partner.

❋ BEING SEX SMART: MINIMIZING THE ODDS OF GETTING INFECTED

If you are not practicing abstinence, the most practical thing you can learn about sexually transmitted diseases is how to most effectively avoid them. So before reading the brief overview of the major STIs in the upcoming pages, you should consider the following ways of minimizing the odds that you'll ever get one.

* **Use a condom and/or other barrier method:** As you saw in Appendix C, male condoms offer the absolute best protection from STIs short of abstinence itself, and thus, until you are in a long-term monogamous relationship with a disease-free partner who himself has already been tested, you should use condoms each and every time you have sex (for more on condoms, see pages 151 and 152). Also, as discussed on page 156, while the female condom is not as effective as the standard male condom against either pregnancy or STIs, it is still an excellent source of protection.

    You should also be aware that some STIs can be transmitted through oral sex. Therefore, you should consider the use of dental dams, which are small latex squares used to cover the female genitals or anal area. Cutting a condom or latex glove and then spreading it open can offer the same level of protection, as can a simple piece of plastic wrap! The basic idea, of course, is that if you completely prevent the exchange of any bodily fluids between you and your partner, you will virtually eliminate the risk of disease transmission, no matter what type of sexual activity you engage in.

* **Communicate honestly with your partner:** For many people, this is easier said than done. But if you aren't able to do it, you shouldn't be having sex anyway, and of course, the same thing goes for your partner! And what should you be talking about? Whether there is any reason to think either of you has been exposed to an STI in the past, and more specifically, whether either of you has any physical symptoms of an STI at present.

    If you or your partner has any unusual symptoms such as genital sores, rash, or discharge, you should have it checked before having sex. Remember that many people have an STI without showing physical symptoms, but observation and discussion can still be helpful in assessing risks and making good decisions.

* **Have yourself tested routinely and practice good hygiene:** If you are sexually active, you and your partner should be examined or tested for STIs periodically, especially when starting a new relationship or whenever you have physical symptoms. Practice good daily hygiene, and remember not to use douches, since your vagina cleans itself!

AIDS/HIV

What it is: AIDS, or acquired immune deficiency syndrome, is caused by HIV, or the human immunodeficiency virus. It is the scariest and most publicized of the STIs, because it can be deadly and has no known cure as of this writing. HIV destroys the body's immune system, which, when healthy, fights off diseases and infections.

How you get it: Through sexual contact with someone who has HIV (unprotected vaginal and anal sex are especially risky). HIV is also spread through blood-to-blood contact by, for example, shared needles.

Symptoms: A person can have HIV within them and still be asymptomatic, not getting actual AIDS for many years. Such people, however, can spread the virus! Once they do get sick, symptoms can include constant fatigue, fever, chills, night sweats, diarrhea, dramatic weight loss, swollen glands, pink or purple blotches on the skin, skin lesions, dry cough, and shortness of breath.

Diagnosis: There are various blood tests available to check for HIV. The decision to get such a test is a serious one that should be discussed with a doctor or clinician first.

Treatment: Although there is no known cure or vaccine as of this writing, there are many drugs that have been developed over the last several years that effectively fight the worst symptoms of the disease.

Long-term consequences: When HIV/AIDS first appeared in the 1980s, almost everybody who got it died within a few years. Today, with the proper drug regimen, diet and other factors, the disease can be managed so that many people can stay alive and healthy, perhaps for decades. Nevertheless, it remains a very dangerous and deadly condition for millions around the world.

Chancroid

What it is: A bacterial infection.

How you get it: Sexual contact with a person who has it, and possibly skin-to-skin contact with a person who has infected sores.

Symptoms: People who have it can be asymptomatic, but more commonly have one of various symptoms, including painful sores around the genitals or anus, as well as painful urination or bowel movements. The sores often have a bad odor.

Diagnosis: A medical exam and blood test.

Treatment: Antibiotics.

Long-term consequences: Without treatment, sores could remain painful indefinitely.

Chlamydia

What it is: A bacterial infection.
How you get it: Sexual contact with someone who has it.
Symptoms: Some people are asymptomatic, though most will have some symptoms, including pelvic pain, painful urination, an unpleasant vaginal discharge, and bleeding after intercourse.
Diagnosis: A medical exam. Usually a urine sample or sample of vaginal discharge is sent to a lab for examination.
Treatment: Antibiotics.
Long-term consequences: If a woman is not treated, she can develop pelvic inflammatory disease, or PID (a severe infection of the reproductive organs), as well as become infertile.

Gonorrhea

What it is: A bacterial infection.
How you get it: Sexual contact with a person who has it.
Symptoms: May be asymptomatic or have various symptoms, including pelvic pain, painful urination, unpleasant vaginal discharge, fever, and sore throat.
Diagnosis: A sample of urine or discharge is examined in a lab.
Treatment: Antibiotics.
Long-term consequences: If not treated, gonorrhea can eventually lead to skin problems, pelvic inflammatory disease (PID), infertility, arthritis, or heart problems.

Hepatitis B

What it is: A liver disease caused by the Hepatitis B virus.
How you get it: Sexual contact with somebody who has it or by sharing contaminated needles, razors, or similar objects with an infected person.
Symptoms: Nausea, fever, abdominal pain, darkened urine, enlarged liver, and jaundice (a yellow discoloration of the eyes and skin). In most cases, these symptoms will disappear within a couple months.
Diagnosis: A blood test.
Treatment: There is no cure, but there are drugs that have shown success in greatly reducing the severity of symptoms. There is also a vaccine that prevents people from getting it.
Long-term consequences: If not treated or managed with drugs, diet, and other strategies, hepatitis B can lead to severe liver damage, liver cancer, and even death.

Herpes

What it is: An infection caused by the herpes simplex virus (HSV).

How you get it: Sexual contact with someone who has herpes, most likely (but not exclusively) when that person has open genital sores. It can also be passed by nonsexual skin-to-skin contact, but this is much rarer.

Symptoms: Painful blisters that break into open sores, usually near the mouth, genital organs, or anus. The sores will dry up and disappear in one to three weeks, but could reappear intermittently every few months. Other symptoms include swollen glands, flu-like symptoms, and fatigue when open sores are present.

Diagnosis: A medical exam of the blisters or sores. A blood test can be performed, as well as a lab examination of the fluid within the sores.

Treatment: There is no known cure (the virus will stay in your body forever), but there are various drugs, creams, and other medicines that can greatly reduce the severity and frequency of open sore outbreaks.

Human Papilloma Virus (HPV or Genital Warts)

What it is: An infection caused by the human papillomavirus (HPV).

How you get it: Sexual or skin-to-skin contact with someone who has it. Being on the Pill puts you at greater risk for acquiring HPV if exposed to an infected partner.

Symptoms: Small, painless cauliflower-like bumps that grow around the sexual organs and anus (some warts may be hidden within the vagina). The bumps may itch and can easily become irritated.

Diagnosis: A medical exam of the bumps, which may include a colposcopy, which utilizes a high-powered microscope (see Glossary). A Pap test may also detect the presence of the virus.

Treatment: There is no known cure (the virus will always stay in your body). However, there are several ways to get rid of the warts themselves, including burning them off with chemicals, electric current, and laser therapy.

Long-term consequences: If not removed, warts can become larger and more difficult to remove. HPV can eventually lead to cervical cancer, and thus needs to be monitored closely over time.

Pubic Lice/Scabies

What it is: Pubic lice (often called "crabs") are parasites that live in pubic hair, while scabies are tiny mites that burrow under the skin, and usually live in the genital area.

How you get it: Mostly by sexual contact with a person who has them, but also by sharing infested towels, bedding, and clothes. Note that condoms will *not* protect against lice and scabies, so if you have any suspicions that your partner has them, you should do a careful visual inspection of their pubic hair. You should be aware that kids in school often get scabies from other kids through completely nonsexual contact.

Symptoms: Both cause extreme itching. If you look very carefully, you will be able to see the lice or eggs in your pubic hair. Scabies cause reddish tracks under the skin in the genital area, as well as in other areas of the body, such as between fingers, in the armpits, and on the feet.

Diagnosis: A visual exam is usually sufficient, though with scabies, it may be necessary to have a microscopic identification of the mites, eggs, larvae, or feces.

Treatment: A variety of lotions and shampoos will eliminate both lice and scabies, but you also will need to wash all clothing and bedding that could be infested in hot soapy water.

Long-term consequences: If not eliminated, the itching may get worse and it could lead to bacterial infections.

Syphilis

What it is: A bacterial infection.

How you get it: Sexual contact with someone who has it.

Symptoms: A painless sore on the mouth, genitals, or anus that will usually go away within a couple weeks.

Diagnosis: A medical exam of the sore or a blood test.

Treatment: Antibiotics.

Long-term consequences: If not treated, a second stage will occur a few months later in which new sores, rash, fever, hair loss, body aches, sore throat, or swollen glands might appear. Eventually those will disappear, but years later a third and final stage can cause severe damage to your heart and brain.

Trichomoniasis

What it is: An infection caused by a parasite.

How you get it: Sexual contact with someone who has it, and in rarer cases, the sharing of damp washcloths, clothes, or towels with someone who has it.

Symptoms: Unpleasant vaginal discharge, painful urination, pain in the lower abdomen, and itching and burning in the genitals.

Diagnosis: A sample of discharge is examined under a microscope.

Treatment: Antibiotics.

Long-term consequences: Without treatment, symptoms could get worse.

Vaginitis

What it is: A vaginal infection caused by yeast, trichomonas, or bacterial vaginosis.

How you get it: Sexual contact with someone who has trichomonas. Note also that these infections can occur without sexual contact, and that certain hormones, antibiotics, and other factors predispose a woman to get a yeast infection.

Symptoms: An unpleasant vaginal discharge as well as vaginal itching or burning, and painful urination.

Diagnosis: A sample of discharge is examined under a microscope.

Treatment: Antibiotics as well as vaginal creams and vaginal suppositories.

Long-term consequences: Without treatment, symptoms could get worse.

HEALTH-RELATED RESOURCES AND BOOKS

❋ ORGANIZATIONS

PLANNED PARENTHOOD FEDERATION OF AMERICA

810 Seventh Avenue
New York, NY 10019
Phone: 1-800-230-7526
Fax: (212) 245-1845
www.plannedparenthood.org
Planned Parenthood is the best known and most important national organization for birth control, abortion, and gynecological services. Their Web site is an excellent resource on where to find and how to contact all of their health clinics throughout the United States.

ALAN GUTTMACHER INSTITUTE

120 Wall Street
New York, NY 10005
Phone: 1-800-355-0244
Fax: (212) 248-1951
E-mail: info@guttmacher.org
www.agi-usa.org
An excellent and reputable organization that specializes in the dissemination of information on STIs, contraceptives, and reproductive health.

AMERICAN COLLEGE OF OBSTETRICIANS AND GYNECOLOGISTS (ACOG)

409 12th Street SW
Washington, DC 20024-2188
Phone: (202) 863-2518
Fax: (202) 484-1595
E-mail: resources@acog.org
www.acog.org
Provides information, including free pamphlets, on contraception, pregnancy, and prenatal care. The above contact info is for their resources center.

SEXUALITY INFORMATION AND EDUCATION COUNCIL
OF THE UNITED STATES (SIECUS)

130 West 42nd Street, Suite #350
New York, NY 10036
Phone: (212) 819-9770
Fax: (212) 819-9776
Email: siecus@siecus.org
www.siecus.org
Premiere national organization devoted to sexuality education and health.

NATIONAL INSTITUTE OF MENTAL HEALTH

Information Resources and Inquiries Branch
5600 Fishers Lane, Room 7C-02
Rockville, MD 20857
Phone: 1-866-615-NIMH (6464)
Fax: (301) 443-4279
Email: nimhinfo@nih.gov
www.nimh.nih.gov
A U.S. government agency devoted to both research and the distribution of information on all types of mental health issues, from anxiety and depression to severe mood swings.

MENTAL HEALTH REFERRALS

Phone: 1-800-THERAPIST, or 1-800-843-7274
Will refer you to a local certified therapist who specializes in your area of need.

EMERGENCY CONTRACEPTIVE HOTLINE

Phone: 1-888-NOT-2-LATE (1-888-668-2528) or 1-800-584-9911

www.NOT-2-LATE.com

Will provide local information on how to obtain the "morning-after pill" if you think you might have become pregnant.

STD (STI) HOTLINE

Phone: 1-800-227-8922

Run by the Centers for Disease Control in Atlanta, Georgia, this hotline is set up to answer questions and provide referrals for all sexually transmitted diseases.

NATIONAL SEXUAL ASSAULT HOTLINE

Phone: 1-800-656-HOPE

www.rainn.org

Counseling, moral support, and information on local rape crisis centers provided by the Rape, Abuse, and Incest National Network.

❋ RECOMMENDED BOOKS

Bell, Ruth, et al. *Changing Bodies, Changing Lives: A Book for Teens on Sex and Relationships.* New York: Times Books, 1998.

Bokram, Karen, et al. *The Girls' Life Guide to Growing Up.* Hillsboro, Oreg.: Beyond Words, 2000.

Drill, Esther, et al. *Deal With It! A Whole New Approach to Your Body, Brain, and Life as a Gurl.* New York: Pocket Books, 1999.

Feinmann, Jane. *Everything a Girl Needs to Know About Her Periods.* Portland, Me.: Ronnie Sellers Productions, 2003.

McCoy, Kathy, et al. *The Teenage Body Book.* New York: Perigee Books, 1999.

Weschler, Toni. *Taking Charge of Your Fertility: The Definitive Guide to Natural Birth Control, Pregnancy Achievement, and Reproductive Health.* New York: HarperCollins, 2006.
  Note: This book is only recommended for women in a long-term monogamous relationship.

Yeager, Selene. *What's Happening to My Body?* New York : Prima Lifestyles, 2002.

Yeager, Selene. *What's with My Body? The Girls' Book of Answers to Growing Up, Looking Good, and Feeling Great.* New York: Prima Lifestyles, 2002.

✳ WEB SITES OF INTEREST

www.cyclesavvy.com
The official web site of this book!

www.4women.gov
Official site of the National Women's Health Information Center.

www.femina.com
A useful gateway site that serves as a comprehensive, searchable directory of links to female-friendly sites and information on the Web.

www.fwhc.org
Official site of the Feminist Women's Health Center, with a huge array of materials on all aspects of female and reproductive health.

www.goaskalice.com
Columbia University's widely used Health Q&A Internet Service created by the Health Education Program of Columbia University.

www.mum.org
Official cyberhome of the Museum of Menstruation and Women's Health. A truly excellent site on the wonders of the female cycle!

www.obgyn.com
A general health site for women and their doctors.

www.scarleteen.com
A well-produced site devoted to all aspects of teen sexuality and sex education.

www.teenwire.com
The official teen site of Planned Parenthood.

www.sxetc.org
A website by teens for teens run by the Rutgers University Network.

www.teenshealth.org
A trendy and cool website that offers comprehensive health advice.

www.gURL.com
A website with honest information about sexuality. Totally girl power!

appendix f

ANSWERS TO
END-OF-CHAPTER
CONFIDENCE BUILDERS

CHAPTER 1—ARE YOU CYCLE LOGICAL? (page12)

1	2	3	4	5		6	7	8	9	10
	P			M						
	R			E			F			
	E			N			A			
	G			O			L			
	N			P			L			
	A			A		E	O		C	
	N			U		G	P		E	
	C		C	S		G	I		R	H
C	Y	C	L	E		S	A	V	V	Y
O		L	E				N	A	I	M
L		I	A				G	X		E
O		T	N				I			N
R		O					N			
		R					A			
		I								
		S								

☐ 9–10 correct Cycle Stoked
☐ 7–8 correct Cycle Choked
☐ 0–6 correct Cycle Croaked

176 Appendix F

✳ CHAPTER 2—TEST YOUR CYCLE SMARTS (page 35)

1) a.   6) a.
2) b.   7) c.
3) b.   8) a.
4) d.   9) c.
5) b.   10) d.

- ☐ 9–10 correct   Cycle Divine
- ☐ 7–8 correct   Cycle Fine
- ☐ 0–6 correct   Cycle Behind

✳ CHAPTER 3—HOW CYCLE WISE ARE YOU? (page 51)

THE VARIABLES THAT CAN:

AFFECT YOUR WAKING TEMPERATURE

- ☐ Drinking alcohol the night before
- ☐ Inconsistent use of electric blanket
- ☐ Less than three hours sleep
- ☐ Taking it later than usual

MASK YOUR CERVICAL FLUID

- ☐ Vaginal infection
- ☐ Sexual arousal fluid
- ☐ Sexual lubricant
- ☐ Spermicides
- ☐ Antihistamines

BE CONSIDERED SECONDARY FERTILITY SIGNS

- ☐ Ovulatory spotting
- ☐ Pain or achiness near the ovaries
- ☐ Fuller vaginal lips than usual

INDICATE A VAGINAL INFECTION

- ☐ Itching, stinging, burning, swelling, or redness
- ☐ Green, foamy, or lumpy discharge
- ☐ The smell of bread baking in your underwear (yeast!)

- ☐ 14–15 correct   Cycle Spiffy
- ☐ 12–13 correct   Cycle Spacey
- ☐ 0–11 correct   Cycle Spazzy

1						P	E	A	**K**						
2						E	V	E	**N**	I	N	G			
3									**O**	T	E	B	O	O	K
4									**W**	E	T				
5						Q	U	A	**L**	I	T	Y			
6									**E**	N	S	A	T	I	O	N
7					B	L	E	E	**D**	I	N	G			
8	O	V	U	L	A	T	I	N	**G**						
9					C	O	V	E	**R**	L	I	N	E		
10					L	U	B	R	**I**	C	A	T	E	D	
11									**S**	T	I	C	K	Y	
12					C	O	M		**P**	L	E	T	E		
13					P	E	R	I	**O**	D					
14									**A**	W	A	K	E	N	I	N	G
15			E	G	G	W	H	I	**T**	E					
16				S	L	I	P	P	E	**R**	Y				

☐ 15–16 correct   Cycle Lucky
☐ 14–13 correct   Cycle Mucky
☐ 11–13 correct   Cycle Sucky
☐ 0–10 correct   Cycle Upchucky

❋ CHAPTER 5—CAN YOU UNRAVEL THE MYSTERIES OF YOUR CYCLE? (page 90)

Words That Do *Not* Belong	Grouping
1. Cervical fluid	Secondary fertility signs
2. While taking vitamins	When spotting may occur
3. Increased intellect	PMS symptoms
4. Clear and slippery secretion	Symptoms of vaginal infection
5. Manicure	Parts of a typical gynecological exam
6. Menstruation	Luteal phase (after ovulation)
7. Drink ice-cold lemonade	Things to do to prevent vaginal infections
8. Toe cramps	Symptoms of a potentially serious pelvic infection
9. Fallopian tubes twisting	Possible causes of ovulatory pain
10. Menstrual elimination	Benefits of charting when you are older

☐ 9–10 correct   Cycle Flow
☐ 7–8 correct   Cycle Slow
☐ 0–6 correct   Cycle No-Go

❋ CHAPTER 6—HOW WILL YOU KNOW WHEN YOU ARE READY FOR SEX? (page 116)

Only the last three questions have correct answers.

What is the one word that should always be at the center of any sexual decision you make?

Respect!

What is the only 100% effective way to prevent an unplanned pregnancy?

Abstinence

What are the four little words that can change your life, and what is the acronym for the fictional radio station that can help you remember them?

Knowledge: Good.
Ignorance: Bad.
KGIB

❋ CHAPTER 7—SOME INTRIGUING QUESTIONS FOR YOU AND YOUR MOM (page 130)

There are no right answers to this one . . . just good communication!

glossary

Abortion

The induced termination of pregnancy before the embryo or fetus is capable of living outside the woman's body.

Abstinence

Avoidance of intercourse. The only foolproof way to avoid pregnancy and sexually transmitted diseases.

Acquired immune deficiency syndrome

See **AIDS**.

AIDS

Acquired immune deficiency syndrome. A fatal disease that is most often transmitted sexually. It is caused by a virus, HIV, that damages the body's immune system, resulting in infections and cancers.

Amenorrhea

Prolonged absence of menstruation. Causes include stress, fatigue, psychological disturbance, obesity, weight loss, anorexia nervosa, hormonal contraceptives, and medical disorders.

Anovulation

The absence of ovulation.

Anovulatory cycle

A cycle in which ovulation does not occur.

Arousal fluid

The colorless, lubricative fluid secreted around the vaginal opening in response to sexual stimulation, in preparation for intercourse. Arousal fluid should not be confused with fertile cervical fluid, which is secreted in a cyclical pattern around ovulation.

Bacteria

Microscopic single-celled organisms. Some types of bacteria live in or on the body without doing any harm and are beneficial to health. Pathogenic bacteria cause disease on entering the body, such as gonococcus, which causes gonorrhea.

Barrier methods of contraception

Any method of contraception that uses a physical barrier to prevent sperm from reaching the ovum, such as a condom or diaphragm.

Bartholin's glands

Two tiny glands, one on each side of the vaginal opening, that produce a thin lubricant when a woman becomes sexually aroused.

Basal body temperature (BBT)

See **Waking temperature.**

BBT

Basal body temperature. See **Waking temperature.**

Biphasic temperature pattern

The pattern on a fertility chart that shows preovulatory low temps followed by postovulatory high temps. The higher postovulatory level lasts for about 12 to 16 days, until the next menstruation. This type of pattern indicates that ovulation has probably occurred (an exception would be in the case of Luteinized Unruptured Follicle Syndrome).

Breakthrough bleeding

Bleeding due to excessive estrogen production, which causes the endometrium to grow beyond the point that it can sustain itself. It usually occurs during anovulatory cycles.

Cervical crypts

Pockets in the lining of the cervix where cervical fluid is produced and that function as temporary shelter for sperm during the woman's fertile phase.

Cervical fluid

The secretion produced within the cervix that acts as a medium in which sperm can travel. Its presence and quality are directly related to the production of estrogen and progesterone. Comparable to a man's seminal fluid, it is one of the two primary fertility signs, along with waking temperature. Cervical fluid typically gets progressively wetter as ovulation approaches. See **Creamy, Eggwhite-quality, Fertile-quality,** and **Sticky cervical fluid.** Often called "cervical mucus."

Cervical mucus

See **Cervical fluid**.

Cervical os

The opening of the cervix, which itself is the lower portion of the uterus that extends into the vagina.

Cervical polyp

An overgrowth of normal tissue that lines the cervical canal, often protruding out of the cervical os. May be asymptomatic or cause spotting or even cramping if it pushes down on the cervix.

Cervical position

The term used to describe an important fertility sign that many women chart when they get older (and which is extensively discussed in the book *Taking Charge of Your Fertility*). It refers to three facets of the cervix: its height, softness, and opening.

Cervical tip

See **Cervical os**.

Cervix

The lower portion of the uterus that projects into the vagina.

Chancre

A small, highly infectious ulcer which is usually painless.

Chancroid

A sexually transmitted infection that causes a painful ulcer at the site of the infection.

Chlamydia

A highly prevalent sexually transmitted disease, which can lead to infertility through scarring of the fallopian tubes.

Clitoris

A small knob of very sensitive erectile tissue. The female counterpart to the tip of the male penis and the center of female sexual pleasure. It is located outside the vagina under a hood of skin at the top of where the labia unite.

Coitus

Sexual intercourse.

Colposcopy

A procedure used to examine the vagina and cervix under magnification through an instrument known as a colposcope. It is of particular value in the early detection of cancer of the cervix.

Conceive

To become pregnant.

Conception

Fusion of the sperm and egg.

Condom

A sheath of thin rubber worn over the penis to prevent conception and the transmission of sexually transmitted infections.

Contraception

The prevention of conception by artificial means.

Contraceptive pill

See **Pill.**

Corpus luteum

The yellow gland formed by the ruptured follicle after ovulation. If an egg is fertilized, the corpus luteum continues to produce progesterone to support the early pregnancy until the placenta is formed. If fertilization does not occur, the corpus luteum degenerates within 12 to 16 days, causing menstruation to occur.

Coverline

A line used to help delineate pre- and postovulatory temperatures on a fertility chart.

Creamy cervical fluid

The cervical fluid quality that is generally wet and often similar to the consistency of hand lotion. It is considered fertile, although not as fertile as the eggwhite-quality cervical fluid that usually follows it.

Cyst

An abnormal saclike structure containing fluid or semisolid material that may be present as a lump in various parts of the body. Most cysts are benign and cause no discomfort, but some may become cancerous.

Depo-Provera

An injectable hormonal contraceptive that lasts for three months.

Diaphragm

A soft rubber device that is inserted in the vagina to cover the cervix and prevent conception. Must be used with a spermicide in order to be effective.

Discharge

A secretion from the vagina. In this book, it always refers to an unhealthy symptom of an infection.

Double ovulation

The release of two separate eggs in one menstrual cycle. Both eggs are released within a 24-hour period, which can lead to fraternal twins if both are fertilized.

Douche

A cleansing fluid that is flushed through the vagina. The practice is unnecessary and strongly discouraged since the normal vaginal environment is altered and the natural self-cleansing mechanism is destroyed.

Dry days

Days when you observe no cervical fluid or bleeding and have a dry vaginal sensation.

Early ovulation

Release of the egg earlier in the cycle than usual or anticipated.

Egg (cell)

See **Ovum.**

Eggwhite-quality cervical fluid

The most fertile type of cervical fluid a woman produces. It typically resembles raw egg-white and tends to be clear, slippery, and stretchy. It usually appears in the two or three days preceding ovulation.

Ejaculation

The release of seminal fluid from the penis during orgasm.

Embryo

The initial stages of development from the fertilized egg to around eight weeks after conception.

Emergency Contraception

See **Morning After Pill**.

Endometrial biopsy

The removal of a small part of the uterine lining (endometrium) for examination under a microscope. Used to determine whether the woman's lining is developing appropriately.

Endometriosis

The growth of endometrial tissue in areas other than the uterus; for example, the fallopian tubes or the ovaries. A woman may not have symptoms or she may have lower abdominal pain that worsens during menstruation, pain during intercourse, and unusually long menstrual periods. Hormone therapy, surgery, and pregnancy may improve the condition. Endometriosis may cause infertility.

Endometritis

An inflammation of the endometrium, or lining of the uterus, usually causing pelvic pain and a thick, unpleasant-smelling yellowish discharge.

Endometrium

The lining of the uterus, which is shed during menstruation. If conception occurs, the fertilized egg implants in it.

Estrogen

The hormone produced mainly in the ovaries responsible for the development of female secondary sex characteristics. It is one of the primary hormones that control the menstrual cycle. Increasing estrogen levels in the first part of the menstrual cycle produces significant changes in the cervical fluid and cervix, indicating fertility.

Estrogenic phase

The estrogen-dominated first phase of the menstrual cycle before ovulation. Also referred to as the follicular phase or preovulatory phase.

Fall-back temperature shift pattern

A type of thermal shift in which the temperature drops on or below the coverline on the second day after having already risen above it.

Fallopian tube

One of a pair of tubes connected to either side of the uterus. Sperm travel up to potentially unite with an egg in the outer third of the tube, after which the fertilized egg is transported toward the uterus through the tube.

False temperature rise

A temperature rise due to causes other than ovulation, such as fever, restless sleep, or drinking alcohol the night before. It is also caused by taking your temperature substantially later than usual.

Female Condom

A polyurethane sheath or pouch that women insert in their vagina as a method of birth control.

Fertile phase

The days of the menstrual cycle during which sexual intercourse or insemination can result in pregnancy.

Fertile-quality cervical fluid

Cervical fluid that is wet, slippery, stretchy, or resembles raw eggwhite. This type of cervical fluid appears around the time of ovulation, allowing sperm to live and travel in it for up to five days.

Fertility

The ability to produce offspring.

Fertility Awareness Method (FAM)

A means of determining your fertility through observing the primary fertility signs of waking temperature and cervical fluid (some women using FAM also observe their cervical position). This method is *not* recommended for teenagers, but it is extensively discussed for post-teen women in the book *Taking Charge of Your Fertility*.

Fertilization

The fusion of a sperm with an egg (ovum), normally in the outer third of the fallopian tube.

Fetus

The developing embryo from about eight weeks after conception until birth.

Fibrocystic breast disease

A misleading term for usually nothing more than a common benign condition characterized by the formation of fluid-filled sacs in one or both breasts.

Fibroid

A fibrous and muscular growth of tissue in or on the wall of the uterus.

Fimbria

The fringed end of the fallopian tube near the ovary. The fimbria, or tendrils of the fringe, pick up the egg shortly after ovulation.

Follicle

A small fluid-filled structure in the ovary that contains the egg (ovum). The follicle ruptures the surface of the ovary, releasing the ovum at ovulation.

Follicle-stimulating hormone (FSH)

The hormone produced by the pituitary gland that stimulates the ovaries to produce mature ova and the hormone estrogen.

Follicular phase

See **Preovulatory phase.**

FSH

See **Follicle-stimulating hormone.**

Fusion

The union of two distinct elements into a whole.

Gamete

The mature reproductive cells of the sperm and ovum.

Genital

Pertaining to the reproductive organs.

Genital contact

Contact between the penis and the vulva without penetration.

Genital herpes

See **Herpes.**

Genitalia (genitals)

The organs of reproduction, especially external.

Genital warts

A sexually transmitted infection, caused by a virus, that leads to small, bumpy warts on the sex organs and anus. See **HPV.**

Gland

Organ that produces chemical substances, including hormones.

Gonads

The primary sex glands of the ovaries and testes.

Gonorrhea

A highly contagious sexually transmitted infection that often causes a thick or yellow vaginal discharge, as well as pain while urinating. If not treated, it can damage the sex organs and lead to infertility.

Gynecologist

A doctor who specializes in women's reproductive health.

HCG

Human chorionic gonadotropin, typically referred to as the "pregnancy hormone." It is produced by the developing embryo when it implants in the uterine lining. Its primary purpose is to maintain the corpus luteum and hence the secretion of estrogen and progesterone until the placenta has developed sufficiently to take over hormonal production. See **Pregnancy test.**

Hepatitis B

A sexually transmitted infection that can cause severe damage to the liver.

Herpes

A common viral infection that is spread by direct skin-to-skin contact. Herpes Simplex Type 1 causes oral herpes (cold sores or fever blisters) and Herpes Simplex Type 2 causes genital herpes (genital sores or sores below the waist). Each type of herpes can be transmitted by simple kissing or vaginal, oral, or anal sex.

HIV

Human immunodeficiency virus. The virus that causes AIDS.

Hormone

A chemical substance produced in one organ and carried by the blood to another organ. An example is FSH, which is produced in the pituitary gland and travels via the blood to the ovary, where it stimulates the growth and maturation of follicles.

HPV (Human Papilloma Virus)

A sexually transmitted infection that can cause small bumpy warts on the sex organs and anus. Often called Genital Warts.

Human chorionic gonadotropin

See **HCG.**

Human immunodeficiency virus

See **HIV.**

Hymen

The thin membrane that protects and partially blocks the entrance of the vagina from birth. May or may not be present in girls, depending on factors such as physical trauma or tampon use.

Hypothalamus

A part of the brain located just above the pituitary gland that controls several functions of the body. It produces hormones that influence the pituitary gland and regulate the development and activity of the ovaries and testes.

Hysterectomy

The surgical removal of the uterus.

Implanon

A contraceptive tube that is inserted in the arm and releases hormones. Lasts up to three years.

Implantation

The process by which the fertilized egg embeds in the uterine lining, or endometrium.

Infertile phases

The phases of the cycle when pregnancy cannot occur. Women usually have both pre-ovulatory and postovulatory infertile phases.

Infertile-quality cervical fluid

A thick, sticky, or opaque-quality cervical fluid that produces a vaginal sensation of dryness or stickiness. It is very difficult for sperm to survive within it.

Infertility

Inability to conceive or maintain a pregnancy, or to provide viable sperm.

Intermenstrual pain

See **Ovulatory pain.**

Intrauterine device

See **IUD.**

IUD (Intrauterine device)

A device placed in the cavity of the uterus to prevent pregnancy. Certain types release hormones while in place.

Kegel exercise

An exercise to contract and relax the vaginal muscles in order to strengthen them. It is also used to help push cervical fluid and semen out of the vaginal opening.

Labia

The two sets of lips surrounding the vaginal opening, forming part of the female external genitalia.

LH

See **Luteinizing hormone.**

Libido

Sexual desire.

Lice

See **Pubic lice/scabies.**

LMP

Abbreviation for "last menstrual period," the first day of the last menstrual period before a pregnancy is suspected or confirmed. The most commonly used means of dating a pregnancy, even though the date of *conception* is more accurate.

Lube

Abbreviation for "lubricative," the slippery vaginal sensation you feel when extremely fertile.

Lubricative sensation

The slippery and wet vaginal sensation you usually feel when fertile-quality cervical fluid is present. Even if no cervical fluid is present, you are still fertile if you have a lubricative sensation!

LUFS (Luteinized Unruptured Follicle Syndrome)

A condition in which the woman's body produces all the signs of ovulation, including a Peak Day and thermal shift, but wihout actually releasing an egg.

Luteal phase

The phase of the menstrual cycle from ovulation to the onset of the next menstruation. It typically lasts from 12 to 16 days, but rarely varies by more than a day or two within an individual woman. Also called the secretory or postovulatory phase.

Luteinized Unruptured Follicle Syndrome

See **LUFS.**

Luteinizing hormone (LH)

A hormone from the pituitary gland that is released in a surge, causing ovulation and development of the corpus luteum.

Menarche

The age at which menstruation begins.

Menopause

The permanent cessation of ovulation, and hence menstruation. A woman is said to have gone through menopause after not having had a period for a full year. It usually occurs when a woman is in her late 40s or early 50s.

Menses

See **Menstruation.**

Menstrual cycle

The cyclical changes in the ovaries, cervix, and endometrium under the influence of the sex hormones. The length of the menstrual cycle is calculated from the first day of menstruation to the day before the following menstruation.

Menstrual cycle, phases of

There are three specific phases in the menstrual cycle:

1. The preovulatory infertile phase, which starts at the onset of menstruation and ends at the onset of the fertile phase.
2. The fertile phase, which includes the days before and after ovulation when intercourse may result in pregnancy.
3. The postovulatory infertile phase, which starts at the completion of the fertile phase and ends at the onset of the next menstruation.

Menstruation

The cyclical bleeding from the uterus as the endometrium is shed. True menstruation is usually preceded by ovulation 12 to 16 days earlier. Day 1 of menstruation is the first day of true red bleeding.

Midcycle pain

See **Ovulatory pain.**

Midcycle spotting

See **Ovulatory spotting.**

Minipill

A type of contraceptive pill that contains an artificial form of progesterone but no estrogen.

Miscarriage

The spontaneous loss of the embryo or fetus from the uterus.

Mittelschmerz

See **Ovulatory pain.**

Monogamous

Having a single sexual partner over an extended period of time.

Monophasic temperature pattern

The pattern on a fertility chart that appears to move randomly up and down, but that does not show preovulatory low temps followed by postovulatory high temps. This type of pattern usually indicates that ovulation has *not* occurred.

Mons pubis

The soft fleshy tissue beneath the pubic hair that protects the internal reproductive organs.

Morning After Pill

An emergency back up pill that greatly reduces the risk of pregnancy if taken within five days after unprotected sex has *already* occurred. It works by keeping the egg from being fertilized by the sperm, or if that fails, by making the endometrial lining of the uterus inhospitable to a fertilized egg.

Mucus

See **Cervical fluid.**

Multiple ovulation

The release of at least two separate eggs in one menstrual cycle. Each of the eggs is released within a 24-hour period of time, which can lead to fraternal twins, triplets, or more if each of the eggs are fertilized.

Nabothian cyst

A harmless cyst on the surface of the cervix.

Natural family planning (NFP)

Method for planning or preventing pregnancy by observation of the naturally occurring signs and symptoms of the fertile and infertile phases of the menstrual cycle. Unlike the Fertility Awareness Method, users of NFP abstain rather than use contraceptive barriers during the fertile phase.

Norplant

A hormonal contraceptive in which six matchstick-sized capsules are inserted just beneath the skin of the upper arm. Lasts for five years. No longer in use. Replaced with the new birth control method called Implanon.

NuvaRing

A small plastic ring which releases contraceptive hormones and is inserted into the vagina, where it stays for three weeks before it is replaced.

Obstetrician

A physician who specializes in pregnancy, labor, and delivery.

OPK

See **Ovulation predictor kits.**

Orgasm

The culmination of sexual excitement in the male or female. Male orgasm is accompanied by ejaculation, the release of seminal fluid from the penis.

Ortho Evra

See **The Patch.**

Ova

Two or more ovum.

Ovarian cyst

A fluid-filled sac that forms on the ovarian wall from a follicle that stops developing before ovulation.

Ovary

One of a pair of female sex organs that produce mature ova, and in turn produce estrogen.

Ovulation

The release of a mature egg (ovum) from the ovary.

Ovulation predictor kit (OPK)

Kit that helps detect the impending release of an egg, usually by testing urine for the presence of luteinizing hormone (LH). The kits are specifically designed to help women get pregnant, but they must never be used as a method of birth control. This is because they only predict ovulation within a day of its occurrence, but sperm can live up to five days or longer in a woman's reproductive tract.

Ovulatory cycle

A cycle in which ovulation occurs.

Ovulatory pain

Lower abdominal pain occurring around the time of ovulation. It is most likely caused by the irritation of the pelvic lining due to a slight amount of blood loss or from the actual breakthrough of the egg through the ovarian wall.

Ovulatory spotting

Light bleeding between two menstrual periods. Usually occurs around the time of ovulation and is often considered a secondary fertility sign.

Ovum

The mature female sex cell, or egg. Analogous to the male sperm.

Patch, The

A thin birth control patch which releases hormones to prevent ovulation. It is changed weekly.

PC muscles

Popular term for the pubococcygeous muscles of the pelvic floor. Their function is to support the bladder, rectum, and uterus.

PCOS

See **Polycystic ovarian syndrome.**

Peak Day

The last day that you produce fertile cervical fluid or have a wet vaginal sensation for any given cycle. It usually occurs either a day before you ovulate or on the day of ovulation itself, and is the most fertile day of the cycle.

Pelvic cavity

The lower portion of the body surrounded by the hips, containing reproductive and other organs.

Pelvic inflammatory disease (PID)

Infection involving inflammation of the internal female reproductive organs, particularly the fallopian tubes and ovaries.

Penis

The external male organ that is inserted into the vagina during intercourse.

Perineum

The membrane between the vulva and the anus that remarkably stretches during childbirth to allow a baby's head to emerge through the vaginal opening.

Period

See **Menstruation.**

PID

See **Pelvic inflammatory disease.**

Pill

Synthetic hormone(s) taken orally to prevent pregnancy. They work by preventing ovulation, changing the cervical fluid to an infertile quality and altering the uterine lining.

Pituitary gland

The master gland at the base of the brain that produces many important hormones, some of which trigger other glands into making their own hormones. The pituitary functions include hormonal control of the ovaries in women and testes in men.

Plan B

See **Morning After Pill.**

PMS

A collection of physical and emotional signs and symptoms that appear during the postovulatory (luteal) phase and disappear at the onset of menstruation. Premenstrual symptoms are experienced by most women in varying degrees.

Polycystic ovarian syndrome (PCOS)

A common endocrine disorder that usually leads to irregular cycles and other hormonal problems, in which developing follicles often remain trapped inside the ovary, later becoming cysts on the internal ovarian wall. Thought to be caused by high blood insulin levels.

Polyp

A soft, fleshy, noncancerous tumor, usually teardrop-shaped, attached to normal tissue by a stem. Often found in the cervix or endometrium.

Postcoital contraception

Emergency contraceptive measure in the form of high-dose pills or insertion of an IUD within a specified time following unprotected intercourse.

Postovulatory phase

See **Luteal phase** and **Menstrual cycle, phases of.**

Preejaculatory fluid

A small amount of lubricating fluid that is emitted from the penis before ejaculation during sexual excitement. May contain sperm.

Pregnancy

The condition of nurturing the embryo or fetus within the woman's body, lasting from conception to birth. Its normal duration is approximately 265 days, though most doctors calculate it from the first day of the last normal period, at approximately 280 days.

Pregnancy test

An urine sample or blood test to determine the presence of human chorionic gonadotropin (HCG), the pregnancy hormone. Blood tests tend to be more sensitive and therefore can be done earlier than a urine test.

Pregnancy wheel

A calculating device used by doctors to determine a pregnant woman's due date. It is based on the assumption that ovulation always occurs on Day 14, and is therefore often inaccurate.

Premenstrual syndrome

See **PMS.**

Preovulatory phase

The variable-length phase of the cycle from the onset of menstruation to ovulation. Also called the follicular phase. See **Menstrual cycle, phases of.**

Progesterone

A hormone produced mainly by the corpus luteum in the ovary following ovulation. It prepares the endometrium for a possible pregnancy. It is also responsible for the rise in basal body (waking) temperature, and for the change in cervical fluid in the postovulatory infertile phase.

Progesterone phase

See **Postovulatory phase.**

Prostaglandin

Any of various fatty acids that are believed to be responsible for severe menstrual cramps.

Pubic lice/scabies

Pubic lice are parasites that live in the public hair, while scabies are tiny mites that burrow under the skin, usually near the genital area. They are both sexually transmitted, though they can also be contracted via nonsexual contact, including from sheets and linens that have been infested.

Puberty

The time of life in boys and girls when the reproductive organs become functional and the secondary sexual characteristics appear.

Pubococcygeous muscles

See **PC muscles**.

Reproductive endocrinologist

A doctor who specializes in reproductive hormones.

Rhythm method

An unreliable method of family planning in which the fertile phase of the cycle is calculated according to the lengths of previous menstrual cycles. Because of its reliance on regular menstrual cycles and long periods of abstinence, it is neither effective nor widely accepted as a modern method of natural family planning.

Rule of Thumb

A guideline in which outlying waking temperatures are ignored, particularly when calculating the coverline.

Scabies

See **Pubic lice/scabies**.

Secondary fertility signs

Physical and emotional changes that may provide supplementary evidence of the fertile phase. Secondary signs include mittelschmerz (ovulatory pain), spotting, and increased sexual feelings.

Secondary sex characteristics

Features of masculinity or femininity that develop at puberty under hormonal control. In the male, this includes deepening voice in addition to the growth of beard, underarm and pubic hair. They are influenced by androgens. In the female, such characteristics include rounding of breasts, waist, and hips, as well as the growth of underarm and pubic hair. They are influenced by estrogens.

Secretory phase

See **Postovulatory phase**.

Semen

The fluid ejaculated from the penis at orgasm. It contains sperm and secretions from the seminal vesicles and prostate gland.

Seminal fluid

See **Semen.**

Sexually transmitted diseases (STDs)

See **Sexually transmitted infections (STIs).**

Sexually transmitted infections (STIs)

Any infection that is transmitted by sexual contact or intercourse.

Short luteal phase

The second phase of the cycle that in some women is deficient in progesterone, typically leading to a phase that is not long enough to allow for successful implantation of a fertilized egg in the uterine wall. A woman usually needs a luteal phase of at least 10 days to sustain a pregnancy.

Slow-rise temperature shift pattern

A type of temperature shift in which temperatures rise by a mere tenth of a degree per day over several days.

Speculum

A two-bladed stainless steel or plastic instrument used to examine the inside of the vagina and the cervix.

Sperm

The mature male sex cell analogous to the female ovum.

Spermicidal

Having sperm-destroying properties.

Spermicides

Vaginal creams, jellies, films, suppositories, or sponges that can immobilize or destroy sperm.

Spinnbarkeit

The stretchy, slippery, and clear quality of cervical fluid that is fertile.

Sponge, The

A soft disposable polyurethane birth control device shaped like a half-dome that contains the spermicide, Nonoxynol-9. It is inserted into the vagina to act as both a barrier and a spermicide.

Spotting

Small amounts of red, pink, or brownish blood occurring during the menstrual cycle.

STDs

Sexually transmitted diseases. The more commonly used term today is sexually transmitted *infections,* or STIs. See **Sexually transmitted infections.**

Sterilization

A procedure that renders an individual permanently unable to reproduce.

Sticky cervical fluid

The type of cervical fluid that often has the texture of library paste or rubber cement. It is usually the first type of cervical fluid that appears in a woman's cycle following menstruation. It is very difficult for sperm to survive in it.

Symptothermal method (STM)

A natural method of family planning combining observation of the basal body (waking) temperature, cervical fluid, and cervical position, along with other secondary fertility signs.

Syphilis

A highly contagious sexually transmitted disease that can eventually lead to extremely serious health consequences if not properly treated.

Temperature chart

A graph showing variation in daily waking temperature reflecting ovulation. See **Biphasic temperature pattern** and **Monophasic temperature pattern.**

Temperature shift

The rise in waking temperature that divides the preovulatory low temperatures from the later postovulatory high temperatures on a biphasic chart. It usually results in temperatures that are at least two-tenths of a degree higher than those of the previous six days.

Testes

Plural of testicle.

Testicle

One of a pair of male sex organs that produce sperm and the male sex hormones (androgens), including testosterone.

Testosterone

A hormone produced by the testes, responsible for the development of male secondary sex characteristics and the functioning of the male reproductive organs.

Thyroid gland

A butterfly-shaped endocrine gland in the lower part of the neck that produces thyroid hormones (including thyroxin) and regulates hormone use and balance in the body.

Today Sponge

See **The Sponge.**

Toxic shock syndrome

A rare but dangerous illness caused by certain powerful bacteria and commonly marked by such symptoms as high fever, vomiting, diarrhea, and severe muscle aches. In the late 1970s, an outbreak of this disease was frequently linked to the use of superabsorbent tampons, but improvement in tampon design makes this much less likely today.

Trichomonas vaginalis

A single-cell protozoan parasite with a whiplike tail that it uses to propel itself through vaginal and urethral mucus.

Trichomoniasis

A very common sexually transmitted infection that is caused by a parasite called trichomonas vaginalis. The most common symptoms are vaginal discharge and pain while urinating.

Tubal Ligation

An operation in which the fallopian tubes are tied or cut so that sperm are blocked from traveling to the egg, and the egg is blocked from traveling on to the uterus. The female equivalent of a vasectomy in men.

Urethra

The tube that carries urine from the bladder to the outside. The female urethra is very short, extending from the bladder to the urinary opening at the vulva. The male urethra is longer, extending along the length of the penis. It also carries the seminal fluid.

Uterus (womb)

The pear-shaped muscular organ in which the fertilized ovum implants and grows for the duration of pregnancy. Muscular contractions of the uterus push the infant out through the birth canal at the time of birth. If implantation does not occur, the uterine lining (endometrium) is shed at menstruation.

Vagina

The muscular canal extending from the cervix to the opening at the vulva, through which menstrual blood leaves the body. Sperm are deposited in the vagina during intercourse. It is also through this birth canal that the baby is delivered during childbirth.

Vaginal discharge

See **Discharge.**

Vaginal infection

An abnormal bacterial or viral growth in the vagina.

Vaginitis

An inflammation of the vagina caused by an infection or other irritation.

Vasectomy

A simple surgical procedure in which the tubes that carry sperm between the testicles and the penis (called the vas deferens) are cut, so sperm cannot get through. The male equivalent of a tubal ligation in women.

VD

Venereal disease. An old-fashioned way of referring to sexually transmitted infections, or STIs.

Venereal disease (VD)

See **Sexually transmitted infections (STIs).**

Vulva

The external female genitalia comprising the clitoris and two sets of vaginal lips.

Vulvodynia

Pain in the vulva, characterized by itching, burning, stinging, or stabbing pain at the opening of the vagina.

Waking temperature

The temperature of the body at rest, taken immediately upon awakening, before any activity. Often referred to as basal body temperature (BBT).

Warts

See **Genital warts.**

Withdrawal

Act of removing the penis from the vagina before ejaculation occurs. Often used as a form of contraception. Although it is not recommended, it is sometimes used in situations when no other contraception is available.

Withdrawal bleeding

Vaginal bleeding resulting from an insufficient level of estrogen to maintain the uterine lining. It usually occurs during anovulatory cycles or during the week in which the contraceptive Pill is not taken.

Womb

See **Uterus.**

Zygote

The fertilized ovum. A single fertilized cell resulting from fusion of the sperm and the egg. After further cell division the zygote is known as a blastocyst, then as an embryo.

Index

luteinizing hormone (LH), 19, 20, 23, *34*
   surge of, 23

males, 15, 58
   double standard and, 102
   fertility of, 11, 45
   preejaculate (precum) of, 99
   sexual experience of, 109–11
   see also penis; sperm
marriage, 113
   as goal, 95, 102
   postponing sex until, 113, 114
masturbation, 106
medical conditions, menstrual irregularities and,
     29
memory loss, 81
menarche, 18
menopause, xvii, 4, 11
menses, *see* menstruation
menstrual cycle, 9, 11, 15–36
   anovulatory, *see* anovulatory cycle
   biology of, 21–27
   defining of, 18
   first day of, 21–23, 141
   frequently asked questions about, 141
   irregular, 28–29
   length of, 18, 20, 21, 25
   pain and, 24, 50, 79–80
   postovulatory (luteal) phase of, 19, 20, 25–28,
     32, 34, 79, 145, 146
   preovulatory (follicular) phase of, 19, 20,
     23–25, 34
   quiz about, 35–36
   support factors and, 18
   uniqueness vs. normalcy and, 126, *126*
menstruation, xv, 8, 10, *31*, 48
   age at start of, 18
   biology of, 21–23, 91
   celebration of, xviii, 21
   cessation of, *see* menopause
   clotting during, 79
   cramps and, xvii, 19, 154
   defining of, 18
   drop in temperature before, 145
   first, xvii, 15, 16, 17
   fun facts about, 18
   getting pregnant and, 141
   gynecological exams during, 87
   heavy, 22
   high waking temperatures and, 145
   hormonal birth control and, 153
   knowledge about, 16

late, xiv, 42
   os and, 7
   prediction of, 74, 75
   surprise, 42, 43
Mental Health Referrals, 172
method failure rate, *see specific kinds of birth control*
midcycle pain, *see* ovulation, pain and
midcycle spotting, 142
Milepristone (RU-486), 160
mirrors, sexual anatomy examined with, 5–7
mittelschmerz, see ovulation, pain and
models, 122–24
money, dating and, 105
Monroe, Marilyn, 124
mons pubis, 8
mood changes and swings, 19, 81
   as birth control side effect, 153, 155, 160
morning-after pill (Plan B), 160
mothers, as fetus, 3, 4
mucus, cervical, *see* cervical fluid
multiple ovulation, 24, 26
mum.org, 174
Museum of Menstruation and Women's Health,
     174

National Institute of Mental Health, 172
National Sexual Assault Hotline, 173
National Women's Health Information Center, 174
natural birth control, xiv, xv, 112
   see also Fertility Awareness Method
nausea, 80, 167
   as birth control side effect, 153, 154, 155, 160
needs, communication of, 107–8
night sweats, 166
nonoxynol-9, 158
NuvaRing, 154

obesity, 29
obgyn.com, 174
open adoption, 97
oral sex, 93, 99, 100, 151, 165
organizations, health-related, 171–73
orgasm, 109, 110
Ortho Evra ("The Patch"), 154
os, *see* cervical os
osteoporosis, 28, 153
outer vaginal lips (labia majora), 5, 6, 8
ova, *see* eggs
ovarian cancer, 155
ovaries, 3, 9, 24
   defining of, *10*
   egg released from, 11, 23, 141

sexually transmitted infections (STIs), 79, 87, 93,
    141, 163–70
    AIDS/HIV, 166
    chancroid, 166
    chlamydia, 100, 167
    genital herpes, 100, 101, 167
    gonorrhea, 167
    hepatitis B, 167
    human papillomavirus, 100, 168
    key facts about, 164
    protection against, 99–101, 111, 112, 149–62,
        163, 164
    pubic lice/scabies, 169
    syphilis, 169
    trichomoniasis, 170
    vaginitis, 170
shaving, of legs, 7
SIECUS (Sexuality Information and Education
    Council of the United States), 172
skin:
    blotches on, 166
    irritation of, 154
sleep, 18
    waking temperature and, 42, 144, 145
"sluts," 102, 103
smoking, birth-control risks and, 154,
    155
sores:
    chancroid and, 166
    herpes and, 168
sore throat, 167
speculums, 87
sperm, 4, 11, 97, 157
    cervical fluid and, 10, 44, 45, 155
    fertilization and, 10, 30, 31, 49
    preejaculate and, 99
    survival of, 10, 30, 99, 112, 141, 161
spermicides, 48, 112, 156, 158
spirituality, 124
sponges, 112, 158
spotting, 77–80
    anovulatory cycle with, 78, 78, 142
    with birth control pills, 78–79
    midcycle, 142
    ovulatory, 24, 50, 77, 77, 142
    premenstrual, 80
STD Hotline, 173
sticky cervical fluid, 45, 45, 47, 61
STIs, see sexually transmitted infections
stress, 28
stroke, 154, 155

swollen glands, 166, 168
syphilis, 169

Taking Charge of Your Fertility (TCOYF)
    (Weschler), ix, xiii, xiv, xv, 129, 161
tampons, 7, 18, 27, 74
    blood clots and, 79
teenwire.com, 174
temperature, waking, *see* waking temperature
temperature chart, *see* charting
thermometers, 55, **58**, 143
Today Sponge, 158
toxic shock syndrome (TSS), 158
travel, 28
trichomoniasis, 170
trust, 107
tubal ligation, 162
twins, 24, 26, 143

ultrasound, 63
underwear, cervical fluid on, 24, 44, 47, *47*, 59
urethra, 7, *9*, 99, 109
    defining of, *8*
urinary tract infections, 156
urination, urine:
    cervical fluid and, 60
    darkened, 167
    pain during, 79, 80, 166, 167, 170
uterus, 7, *9*, 49
    cross-section of, *10*
    defining of, *10*
    fertilized egg in, 30, *31*
    gynecological exam and, 86, 87
    IUD and, 157
    lining of, *see* endometrium
    purpose of, 9
    tip forward of, *9*

vagina, 7, *9*, 23, 97
    color of, 5
    defining of, *8*, *10*
    dryness of, 153
    functions of, 5, *8*, *10*
    gynecological exam and, 86–87
    hygienic efficiency of, 118, 165
    hymen in, 7
    irritation of, 154, 158
    itching of, 49, 75, 170
    muscularity of, 7
    penis compared with, 4
    survival of sperm in, 45

My Age _____ Month _____ Year _____ Fertility Cycle # _____ This cycle length _____

Cycle Day	1	2	3	4	5	6	7	8	9	10	11	12	13	14	15	16	17	18	19	20	21	22	23	24	25	26	27	28	29	30	31	32	33	34	35	36	37	38	39	40
Date																																								
Day																																								

Waking Temperature

(degree scale rows: 7 6 5 4 3 2 1 / 98 / 9 8 7 6 5 4 3 2 1 / 97 repeated across all 40 cycle-day columns)

Temp Count for Luteal Phase																																								

Cycle Day	1	2	3	4	5	6	7	8	9	10	11	12	13	14	15	16	17	18	19	20	21	22	23	24	25	26	27	28	29	30	31	32	33	34	35	36	37	38	39	40
Period, Spotting, & Peak Day																																								
Vaginal Sensation — Dry, Sticky, Damp, Wet, Lube																																								
Cervical Fluid Description																																								
Quantity — Scant, Moderate, A lot																																								
Color — White, Yellow, Streaked, Clear																																								
Consistency — Dry, Sticky, Crumbly, Creamy, Wet, Slippery, Stretchy																																								

Cycle Day	1	2	3	4	5	6	7	8	9	10	11	12	13	14	15	16	17	18	19	20	21	22	23	24	25	26	27	28	29	30	31	32	33	34	35	36	37	38	39	40

Notes

(Cycle Day 7 column: BSE)

My Age _____   Month _____   Year_____   Fertility Cycle #_____   This cycle length _____

Cycle Day	1	2	3	4	5	6	7	8	9	10	11	12	13	14	15	16	17	18	19	20	21	22	23	24	25	26	27	28	29	30	31	32	33	34	35	36	37	38	39	40
Date																																								
Day																																								

Waking Temperature (gradations from 97 to 98 degrees, each column marked 7 6 5 4 3 2 1 / 98 / 9 8 7 6 5 4 3 2 1 / 97)

| Temp Count for Luteal Phase | | | | | | | | | | | | | | | | | | | | | | | | | | | | | | | | | | | | | | | | |

Cycle Day	1	2	3	4	5	6	7	8	9	10	11	12	13	14	15	16	17	18	19	20	21	22	23	24	25	26	27	28	29	30	31	32	33	34	35	36	37	38	39	40
Period, Spotting, & Peak Day																																								

Vaginal Sensation
Dry, Sticky, Damp, Wet, Lube

Cervical Fluid Description

Quantity
Scant, Moderate, A lot

Color
White, Yellow, Streaked, Clear

Consistency
Dry, Sticky, Crumbly
Creamy, Wet, Slippery, Stretchy

Cycle Day	1	2	3	4	5	6	7	8	9	10	11	12	13	14	15	16	17	18	19	20	21	22	23	24	25	26	27	28	29	30	31	32	33	34	35	36	37	38	39	40

Notes

(Day 7: BSE)

Stressed Out																																								
Feeling Blue																																								
Moody																																								
Excited																																								
Crampy																																								
Bloated																																								
Tender Breasts																																								
Chocolate Cravings																																								